Clinical Pearls in
PULMONOLOGY

Clinical Pearls in PULMONOLOGY

Hemanth IK MBBS MD
Associate Professor
Deparment of Internal Medicine
KMCT Medical College
Kozhikode, Kerala, India

Co-author
Binuraj C MBBS MD DTCD
Associate Professor
Department of Chest Medicine
KMCT Medical College
Kozhikode, Kerala, India

Foreword
MC Vinod Krishnan

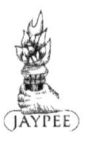

The Health Sciences Publisher
New Delhi | London | Panama

Jaypee Brothers Medical Publishers (P) Ltd

Headquarters
Jaypee Brothers Medical Publishers (P) Ltd
4838/24, Ansari Road, Daryaganj
New Delhi 110 002, India
Phone: +91-11-43574357
Fax: +91-11-43574314
Email: jaypee@jaypeebrothers.com

Overseas Offices

J.P. Medical Ltd
83 Victoria Street, London
SW1H 0HW (UK)
Phone: +44 20 3170 8910
Fax: +44 (0)20 3008 6180
Email: info@jpmedpub.com

Jaypee-Highlights Medical Publishers Inc
City of Knowledge, Bld. 235, 2nd Floor, Clayton
Panama City, Panama
Phone: +1 507-301-0496
Fax: +1 507-301-0499
Email: cservice@jphmedical.com

Jaypee Brothers Medical Publishers (P) Ltd
17/1-B Babar Road, Block-B, Shaymali
Mohammadpur, Dhaka-1207
Bangladesh
Mobile: +08801912003485
Email: jaypeedhaka@gmail.com

Jaypee Brothers Medical Publishers (P) Ltd
Bhotahity, Kathmandu
Nepal
Phone: +977-9741283608
Email: kathmandu@jaypeebrothers.com

Website: www.jaypeebrothers.com
Website: www.jaypeedigital.com

© 2017, Jaypee Brothers Medical Publishers

The views and opinions expressed in this book are solely those of the original contributor(s)/author(s) and do not necessarily represent those of editor(s) of the book.

All rights reserved. No part of this publication may be reproduced, stored or transmitted in any form or by any means, electronic, mechanical, photocopying, recording or otherwise, without the prior permission in writing of the publishers.

All brand names and product names used in this book are trade names, service marks, trademarks or registered trademarks of their respective owners. The publisher is not associated with any product or vendor mentioned in this book.

Medical knowledge and practice change constantly. This book is designed to provide accurate, authoritative information about the subject matter in question. However, readers are advised to check the most current information available on procedures included and check information from the manufacturer of each product to be administered, to verify the recommended dose, formula, method and duration of administration, adverse effects and contraindications. It is the responsibility of the practitioner to take all appropriate safety precautions. Neither the publisher nor the author(s)/editor(s) assume any liability for any injury and/or damage to persons or property arising from or related to use of material in this book.

This book is sold on the understanding that the publisher is not engaged in providing professional medical services. If such advice or services are required, the services of a competent medical professional should be sought.

Every effort has been made where necessary to contact holders of copyright to obtain permission to reproduce copyright material. If any have been inadvertently overlooked, the publisher will be pleased to make the necessary arrangements at the first opportunity.

Inquiries for bulk sales may be solicited at: jaypee@jaypeebrothers.com

Clinical Pearls in Pulmonology
First Edition: **2017**
ISBN 978-93-5152-417-5

Dedicated to

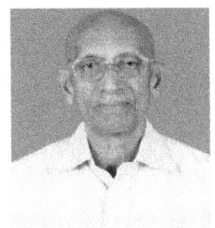

*My grandfather Dr TK Sudhakaran,
whose life as a doctor has inspired me
to take up this noble profession*

Foreword

In this era of technology, there is a general feeling that investigative medicine is going to replace the age-old bedside clinical medicine; however, anybody with at least a few years of experience in medical profession knows otherwise. A good history with thorough clinical examination will clinch the diagnosis in most of the patients. This not only saves the cost and pain of unnecessary investigations but also helps in building a good doctor–patient relationship.

There are so many good textbooks on clinical medicine that are time tested and followed by generations of medical students. Why take the trouble of bringing out one more? This is probably the question everybody asked when they came to know that Dr Hemanth IK has written a textbook on clinical medicine. When they see his work they will know why it is worthwhile to have one more.

It is well known that in medicine and probably in all subjects, it is easy to ask questions but difficult to get the right answer. This probably inspired the author to present the subject in a totally different way. Although the questions and answers method of presenting the subject is not a new one, there are very few good books that are written in this way, especially in clinical medicine. The book is also well illustrated. The students will definitely find this very useful, especially when it comes to answering tough questions during their clinical and oral examinations.

I strongly recommend this book to all the undergraduate students of medicine. The junior residents also will find this book useful. Presently, this book covers only the respiratory system and I am sure that Dr Hemanth IK will bring out many more books in different clinical specialties of internal medicine in the near future. I congratulate him for his effort and wish him good luck.

MC Vinod Krishnan MBBS MD
Professor and Head
Department of Medicine
KMCT Medical College
Kozhikode, Kerala, India

Preface

The importance of clinical medicine appears to be on the downfall with most of the modern textbooks giving more importance to the investigative part of medicine. But in country like India, where majority of the population reside in the rural areas with very little laboratory facilities, it is essential that we should concentrate on the clinical side of medicine. This book has been written keeping this aspect in mind. To make things more interesting, the facts are presented in a questions and answers format. I sincerely hope that my humble attempt will be beneficial to all of you.

I am extremely thankful to Dr Binuraj C, who has helped me in editing this book and his suggestions were very valuable. I am also thankful to Professor MC Vinod Krishnan, who has taken all the pains to go through the matter, and his suggestions were of immense help in writing this book.

I am also thankful to Shri Jitendar P Vij (Group Chairman) and Mr Ankit Vij (Group President) of M/s Jaypee Brothers Medical Publishers (P) Ltd, New Delhi, for helping me to bring out this book.

I am thankful to all my teachers, collegues and well wishers, for their support given to me.

Hemanth IK

Contents

CHAPTER 1. History and General Examination 1
CHAPTER 2. Inspection and Palpation of the Chest Wall 43
CHAPTER 3. Chest Percussion 59
CHAPTER 4. Auscultation of the Chest 79
CHAPTER 5. Interstitial Lung Diseases 98
CHAPTER 6. Tuberculosis 104
CHAPTER 7. Bronchiectasis 119
CHAPTER 8. Pneumonia 125
CHAPTER 9. Diseases of the Airways and Lung Vasculature 134
CHAPTER 10. Radiology 146

Index *163*

Chapter
1

History and General Examination

1. What are the characteristics of pleuritic type of chest pain?

Pleuritic chest pain is due to the inflammation of the pleura secondary to infection, inflammation or infarction of the adjacent pulmonary parenchyma. Primary tumors like mesothelioma or metastasis from the lung, breast, ovary, etc. may involve the parietal pleura and cause pleuritic pain.

Pleuritic pain is exacerbated by movements like deep inspiration and coughing. The pain forces the patient to hold his breath at some point during inspiration and hence there is shallow breathing. The patient prefers to lie down on the affected side so as to reduce the chest movements. When the central portion of the diaphragmatic parietal pleura is irritated, pain may be referred to the ipsilateral shoulder or neck region.

Chest wall pain can sometimes mimic pleuritic pain as in Coxsackie B virus infection. This infection causes pleurodynia (Bornholm disease or "Devil's grip" or Epidemic myalgia) and the patient has severe myalgia of the intercostal muscles (Box 1.1).

> **Box 1.1:** Pathways of pain sensation
> - Chest wall via the intercostal nerves
> - Parietal pleura via the intercostal nerves
> - Diaphragmatic pleura via the phrenic nerve
> - Bronchial tree and pulmonary vasculature via the vagus nerve
> - Lung interstitium via the vagus nerve

It has to be remembered that even in the absence of involvement of the parietal pleura, lung tumors can produce a visceral pain syndrome. It is postulated that this pain syndrome is mediated via the vagal afferent neurons.

2. What is meant by precordial catch syndrome?

Precordial catch syndrome (also known as Texidor's twinge) is a common cause of chest pain in children, adolescents and young adults. It manifests itself as a very intense, sharp pain, typically at the left side of the chest. Episodes of pain occur most often at rest, while sitting or lying down. The pain typically lasts from 30 seconds to a few minutes and it does not radiate. Breathing in, and sometimes breathing out, often intensifies the pain. On some occasions, breathing in or out suddenly will cause a small popping or cracking sensation in the chest, which results in the disappearance of pain. The cause of pain is unknown, and in most cases, the pain is resolved quickly and completely. There is no role for any form of medication.

3. How will you classify respiratory failure?

Respiratory failure is defined as respiratory dysfunction resulting in abnormalities of oxygenation or ventilation severe enough to threaten the function of vital organs. The major clinical sign of respiratory failure is cyanosis.

Respiratory failure can arise from an abnormality in any of the "effector" components of the respiratory system, i.e. (1) central nervous system, (2) peripheral nervous system, (3) respiratory muscles and chest wall, (4) airways and (5) alveoli. The central and peripheral nervous systems, respiratory muscles and chest wall, and the airways together constitute the "respiratory pump". Hypercapnia is the hallmark of respiratory pump failure, whereas hypoxemia indicates a primary disturbance in alveolar function (Table 1.1).

Table 1.1: Types of respiratory failure

Type I failure		Type II failure
Hypoxemia without hypercapnia (↑ PAO_2–PaO_2 gradient)		**Hypoxemia with hypercapnia**
CXR showing infiltrates	No infiltrates on the CXR	• Chronic bronchitis
• Cardiac failure • ARDS • Pneumonia • Interstitial lung disease	• Pulmonary embolism • Emphysema • Acute airway obstruction • Intracardiac shunt	• Neuromuscular disorders

4. What are the clinical features of hypercapnia?

The chief symptoms of hypercapnia ($PaCO_2$ more than 50 mm Hg) are dyspnea and headache. The important signs are tachypnea, tachycardia, warm peripheries with bounding pulses, hypertension, conjunctival hyperemia, asterixis (flapping tremor), myoclonus and papilledema. Papilledema is due to increased intracranial pressure secondary to cerebral vasodilation (Box 1.2).

> **Box 1.2:** Signs of hypercapnia
>
> - Tachypnea and tachycardia
> - Warm peripheries with bounding pulse
> - Conjunctival hyperemia
> - Asterixis and myoclonus
> - Hypertension
> - Papilledema

With worsening hypercapnia, the patient can become increasingly confused, somnolent and obtunded. This condition is referred to as carbon dioxide narcosis. It has to be remembered that cyanosis is a sign of hypoxemia and not hypercapnia. So presence of cyanosis in a patient with "respiratory pump" failure indicates severe hypoventilation with mixed hypercapnia and hypoxemia.

5. **What is chronic cough?**

   Cough is an explosive expiration that clears and protects the airways. It is caused by the stimulation of vagal afferents in the intrapulmonary airways, the larynx or the pharynx (the cough center is located in the medulla). Chronic cough is a cough that lasts for a duration of eight weeks or more.

6. **What is postural cough and what are the causes of chronic cough?**

   A cough induced by postural change suggests chronic lung abscess, cavitary TB, bronchiectasis or a pedunculated tumor. The most common causes of chronic cough are the following:
   - Postnasal drip syndrome (PNDS)
   - Gastroesophageal reflux (GERD)
   - Pulmonary tuberculosis
   - Smoking and other irritants
   - Chronic bronchitis and bronchial asthma
   - Drugs like ACE inhibitors

Chronic bronchitis is a condition where there is cough with sputum production on most days for a period of three consecutive months for two successive years. The common complications of chronic cough are the following:
- Rib fracture
- Pneumothorax
- Abdominal wall hernias
- Cough syncope

In cough syncope, a bout of cough produces increased intrathoracic pressure. This leads to a decrease in the cardiac output and cerebral perfusion. This results in the syncopal attack.

7. What are the differences between hemoptysis and hematemesis?

Hemoptysis is defined as the expectoration of blood or blood-streaked sputum that originates below the level of the vocal cords (bleeding originating above the vocal cords is called as spurious hemoptysis). Hematemesis is defined as the vomiting of blood from the upper gastrointestinal tract (Table 1.2).

Table 1.2: Difference between hemoptysis and hematemesis

Hemoptysis	Hematemesis
Preceded by bouts of coughing	Preceded by nausea
Contents are bright red in color	Contents are dark brown in color
Contents are alkaline	Contents are acidic
Contents are frothy	Contents mixed with food particles
Past history of lung diseases (e.g. tuberculosis, bronchiectasis)	Past history of gastrointestinal diseases (e.g. cirrhosis, peptic ulcer)

8. What is meant by melanoptysis?

Melanoptysis is the expectoration of black colored sputum. It is seen in the complicated form of coal worker's pneumoconiosis known as progressive massive fibrosis (PMF). Patients with bronchopulmonary aspergillosis may also bring up black sputum or sputum with black parts in it. The black part in the sputum is the fungal element of aspergillus.

9. What is meant by aspergilloma?

Aspergilloma is a mass of fungal hyphae within pre-existing lung cavities (almost always in the upper lobes). The major symptoms include massive hemoptysis, cough, low grade fever and weight loss. Chest X-ray and CT scan shows a meniscus of air around the fungal ball. Surgical therapy of aspergilloma has high morbidity and mortality. An alternative therapeutic option is the intracavitary instillation of the antifungal amphotericin.

10. What is the most common cause for hemoptysis?

Pulmonary infection is the most common cause of hemoptysis, accounting for 60–70% of cases. Infection causes superficial mucosal inflammation and edema that can lead to the rupture of the superficial blood vessels.

Invasive bacteria (e.g. *Staphylococcus aureus, Pseudomonas aeruginosa)* or fungi (e.g. *Aspergillus species*) are the most common infectious causes of hemoptysis. Viruses such as influenza also may cause severe hemoptysis. HIV infection predisposes the patients to several conditions that can produce hemoptysis, including pulmonary Kaposi's sarcoma.

11. What is massive hemoptysis and what are the common causes for recurrent hemoptysis?

The lungs are supplied with dual modes of circulation. The pulmonary arterial circulation arises from the right ventricle and is a low pressure system supplying the pulmonary parenchyma. The bronchial artery circulation arises from the aorta and is a high pressure system supplying the airways.

Eventhough the bronchial artery circulation constitutes only 2% of the total pulmonary circulation, it is a high pressure system. So bleeding from the tributaries of this circulation can be massive. Massive hemoptysis is the expectoration of more than 600 mL of blood in 24 hours (*Ref: The Washington Manual of Medical Therapeutics, 33rd edition*). Bronchial arterial bleeding occurs in chronic bronchitis, bronchiectasis, malignancies, broncholithiasis and with the presence of foreign bodies in the airways. Recurrent hemoptysis can occur in the following conditions.

- Bronchiectasis
- Bronchial tumors (adenomas or carcinomas)
- Recurrent small pulmonary emboli with infarction
- Pulmonary arteriovenous malformation
- Cavitary lung disease (TB, aspergilloma, etc.)

12. What are the mechanisms of hemoptysis in pulmonary tuberculosis?

Pulmonary tuberculosis is one of the common causes for hemoptysis. The various mechanisms of hemoptysis in pulmonary tuberculosis are the following:

- Congestion or hyperemia of the bronchial mucus membrane leading to hemorrhage from the poorly supported capillaries

- Erosion of the walls of blood vessels (pulmonary veins, bronchial arteries) by the granulomatous tissue
- Rupture of Rasmussen's aneurysm
- Dislodgement of calcareous masses (broncholith) from healed cavities leads to the rupture of adjacent capillaries.

Thus in pulmonary tuberculosis, blood vessels supplied by both modes of circulation (bronchial and pulmonary arterial) are involved in the causation of hemoptysis. So massive hemoptysis can sometimes occur in pulmonary tuberculosis.

13. What are the various factors that influence the color of the sputum?

Phlegm or mucus produced from the lower respiratory tract is often combined with saliva and secretions from the nose and the pharynx to form sputum. Normally the sputum is swallowed and approximately 30 mL of airway mucus is eliminated by the gastrointestinal tract daily.

Sputum due to chronic irritation of the bronchi in conditions like chronic bronchitis is usually white or mucoid. If there is infection, the sputum turns yellow due to the presence of leukocytes and this yellow sputum may turn to green by the action of the enzyme verdoperoxidase. However, yellow sputum in bronchial asthma can be caused by the presence of eosinophils even in the absence of infection. Pink frothy sputum due to the admixture of blood and air is seen in pulmonary edema. Sticky and "rusty" sputum due to uniform dispersion of blood in the sputum is characteristic of lobar pneumonia. Red currant jelly sputum is seen in pneumonia due to *Klebsiella*. "Anchovy sauce" sputum is seen in amebic lung abscess (Table 1.3).

Condition	Color of sputum
White or mucoid	Chronic bronchitis
Yellow	Pulmonary infections
Pink	Acute pulmonary edema
Rusty	Lobar pneumonia
Red currant jelly	*Klebsiella pneumoniae*
Anchovy sauce	Pulmonary amebiasis

Table 1.3: Color of sputum

14. What is dyspnea?

The American Thoracic Society defined dyspnea as " a subjective experience of breathing discomfort consisting of qualitatively distinct sensations that vary in intensity." The sensation of dyspnea originates in the cerebral cortex in response to stimuli arising from receptors in the lungs (e.g. J receptors), upper airways and the respiratory muscles.

15. What is meant by paroxysmal nocturnal dyspnea (PND)?

Paroxysmal nocturnal dyspnea or PND is a type of breathlessness that wakes up the patient from sleep at midnight. It indicates left ventricular dysfunction. Typically, the patient suddenly gets up from sleep and walks to the window to breathe in fresh air, and it takes several minutes for relief of dyspnea to occur.

PND is caused by pulmonary congestion during recumbency. In the horizontal position there is redistribution of blood volume from the lower extremities and splanchnic beds to the lungs. In normal individuals this redistribution has little effect. But in patients with left ventricular dysfunction, this additional blood volume cannot be pumped out by the failing left ventricle. This results in pulmonary venous congestion producing dyspnea.

16. What are the causes of acute onset of dyspnea?

Acute dyspnea is defined as dyspnea arising in the previous 24–48 hours. The most common etiologies are the following and there is a rule of 10 Ps to remember them (Box 1.3).

Box 1.3: Rule of 10 Ps

1. Peanut or other foreign body inhalation
2. Pneumothorax
3. Pulmonary embolism
4. Pump failure or acute left ventricular failure
5. Pulmonary constriction or asthma
6. Pericardial tamponade
7. Pneumonia
8. Peak seekers or high altitude sickness
9. Psychogenic
10. Poisons or drugs

Some of the above causes produce sudden (i.e. within minutes) onset of dyspnea. Pneumothorax, pulmonary embolus, foreign body inhalation and acute left ventricular failure can result in the sudden onset of dyspnea.

17. What are the clinical presentations of pulmonary embolism?

In pulmonary embolism, the embolus usually originates from the deep veins of the legs, most commonly the calf veins. Most patients present with either one or more of the following typical syndromes of pulmonary embolism, as follows:

- The "pleuritic pain/hemoptysis syndrome" is usually due to pulmonary infarction secondary to recurrent small pulmonary emboli.
- The "uncomplicated dyspnea syndrome" occurs in patients with submassive pulmonary embolism who do not develop pulmonary infarction.
- The "circulatory collapse syndrome" occurs in patients with acute cor pulmonale due to massive pulmonary embolism. These patients usually have hypotension. This may produce an S wave in lead I and a Q wave in lead III. T wave inversion in lead III may also be present, producing the well known S1, Q3, T3 pattern (seen rarely in only about 10% of patients). Sinus tachycardia is the most common Electrocardiography (ECG) finding in pulmonary embolism (Fig. 1.1).

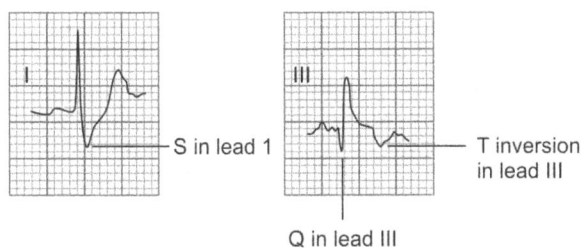

Fig. 1.1: ECG showing S1, Q3, T3 pattern

18. What is the difference between orthopnea, trepopnea and platypnea?

Orthopnea is dyspnea in the supine posture. Orthopnea is caused by pulmonary congestion during recumbency. It occurs in those with congestive heart failure, bilateral diaphragmatic paralysis, severe COPD and obstructive sleep apnea. The severity of orthopnea can be clinically graded by the number of pillows the patient uses before feeling comfortable (i.e. two or three pillow orthopnea).

Trepopnea is dyspnea in the lateral decubitus posture. It occurs in unilateral lung collapse due to either an endobronchial obstructive lesion or massive pleural effusion. In these situations, the patient feels better and has improved oxygenation with the good lung in the dependent position. Platypnea is dyspnea in the upright posture. It is seen in conditions where the lower lobes are affected more than the upper lobes. So, the patient is comfortable in the supine position which decreases the perfusion to the diseased lower lobes. It is seen in hepatopulmonary syndrome, left atrial myxoma, etc.

19. What are the pulmonary causes for dyspnea without much clinical signs on examination of the respiratory system?

The important pulmonary causes for dyspnea without much clinical signs on examination of the respiratory system are the following:
- Hyperventilation syndrome
- Small pulmonary infarctions due to multiple small pulmonary emboli
- Early interstitial lung disease

The only physical sign in all the three conditions is usually tachypnea. Another important cause for dyspnea without much cardiorespiratory signs is metabolic acidosis in conditions like diabetic ketoacidosis, chronic renal failure, etc.

20. What are the peculiarities of a "blue bloater"?

In advanced COPD, two symptom patterns tend to emerge and they are historically referred to as "blue bloaters" and "pink puffers". However, most COPD patients have evidence of both patterns in varying proportions. In those with predominant chronic bronchitis, the main defect is hypoventilation of the lungs. The pulmonary capillary bed is relatively undamaged, and so the perfusion is fairly normal. The body tries to compensate the hypoventilation by increasing the perfusion through the lungs. This results in rapid circulation through a poorly ventilated lung.

This combination of hypoventilation and increased perfusion leads to hypoxia, severe hypercapnia, respiratory acidosis, secondary polycythemia, pulmonary artery vasoconstriction and cor pulmonale. These people are referred to as "blue bloaters" and their major symptom is chronic productive cough with mild dyspnea.

21. What are the peculiarities of a "pink puffer"?

In those with predominant emphysema, there is destruction of the pulmonary capillary bed in the alveolar septa. So lung perfusion is affected to a greater extent than ventilation. The body tries to compensate this underperfusion by hyperventilating the lungs. So there is limited blood flow through a fairly well-ventilated lung.

This combination of underperfusion and hyperventilation leads to severe hypoxia. The extreme hyperventilation leads to pulmonary cachexia characterized by muscle wasting and weight loss. They are referred to as "pink puffers" and their major symptom is severe dyspnea with occasional rare cough. Cyanosis is usually absent in the early stages.

22. What are the differences between centriacinar and panacinar emphysema?

In centriacinar emphysema, the proximal parts of the acini are mostly involved. This type of emphysema is the commonest pattern that occur in chronic smokers. The lesions are common in the upper lobes.

In panacinar emphysema, both the proximal and distal parts of the acini are involved uniformly. It is the commonest pattern occurring in alpha-1 antitrypsin deficiency. The lesions are common in the lower lobes (Table 1.4).

Table 1.4: Types of emphysema

Centriacinar emphysema	Panacinar emphysema
Seen in smokers	Seen in alpha-1 antitrypsin deficiency
Upper lobes commonly involved	Lower lobes commonly involved
Proximal parts of acini are affected	Proximal and distal parts of acini affected

23. What is cough variant asthma?

Coughing is the only clinical manifestation of asthma in up to 50% of patients with asthma. This type of asthma is referred to as cough variant asthma. Cough variant asthma should be considered when persistent cough is exacerbated by cold or exercise or when cough worsens at night. Airway hyper-responsiveness may also suggest the diagnosis of cough variant asthma. This disease responds to asthma medications such as bronchodilators and inhaled corticosteroids.

24. What is occupational asthma?

Occupational asthma is now the most common form of occupational respiratory disorder. It accounts for about 5% of all adult onset asthma cases. This should be considered in all adult asthmatics of working age group, particularly if symptoms improve during the time away from the workplace (i.e. weekends or holidays). Atopic individuals and smokers appear to be at increased risk. Byssinosis is an asthma like occupational lung disease seen in cotton textile workers. It is caused by inhalation of cotton dust.

25. What is silent chest?

Silent chest is seen in very severe asthma due to **severe airflow limitation.** Here the airflow rate is below the critical level necessary to generate wheezing. So, the chest appears to be silent in spite of the severe bronchospasm. The only diagnostic clue on auscultation may be the globally diminished vesicular breath sounds with prolonged expiration.

26. How will you distinguish bronchial asthma from cardiac asthma?

Cardiac asthma is the clinical manifestation of paroxysmal nocturnal dyspnea which occurs secondary to intra-alveolar edema in left ventricular dysfunction. This intra-alveolar edema causes congestion of the bronchial mucosa which leads to asthmatic attack. The typical attack of dyspnea of cardiac asthma occurs at one or two o'clock in the morning, awakening the patient after 2 to 4 hours of sound sleep. Shortness of breath, wheezing and a sense of a weight on the chest, forces the patient to sit up in bed. Often the attack is relieved in a few minutes by coughing up of frothy sputum or with diuretics (here dypnea preceeds cough). The patient then returns to sleep for the remainder of the night. The patient usually has other clinical evidences of pre-existing cardiac or renal disease (like S3, cardiomegly).

Bronchial asthma is characterized by episodic reversible bronchial obstruction due to the hyper-responsiveness of the tracheobronchial tree to a variety of intrinsic and extrinsic stimuli. Patients with bronchial asthma are awakened usually at 3 or 4 o'clock in the morning with cough, wheezing and dyspnea and this is followed by expectoration of copious amount of tenacious mucus (here cough preceeds dyspnea). The attack is usually relieved by parentral or inhaled bronchodilators (Table 1.5).

Table 1.5: Differences between cardiac and bronchial asthma

Cardiac asthma	Bronchial asthma
Occurs around midnight	Occurs in early morning hours
Dyspnea precedes cough	Cough precedes dyspnea
Relieved with diuretics	Relieved with bronchodilators

It is very difficult to differentiate between cardiac asthma and bronchial asthma as a cause of dyspnea, wheezing and coughing in elderly patients because many of the symptoms of one condition are also the symptoms of the other. Recent studies have suggested that an increased serum level of brain natriuretic peptide (>100 pg/mL) differentiates dyspnea due to heart failure from that due to pulmonary dysfunction.

27. **What are the common causes of hoarseness of voice?**
Hoarseness is commonly caused by acute laryngitis due to upper respiratory infection or vocal overuse.

Both the above conditions are self-limiting. Persisting hoarseness suggests gastroesophageal reflux disease, chronic vocal overuse, tobacco exposure, benign vocal-fold nodules, hypothyroidism, laryngeal carcinoma, recurrent laryngeal nerve injury or infiltrative diseases such as amyloidosis or sarcoidosis.

28. **What are the anatomical pecularities of recurrent laryngeal nerve?**

    The larynx serves four important functions (breathing, swallowing, coughing and phonation) that require an intact recurrent laryngeal nerve. The axons of the recurrent laryngeal nerve travel with the vagus nerve in the neck. In the superior mediastinum, the left recurrent laryngeal nerve loops around the aorta, ascends within the tracheoesophageal groove, and then enters the larynx. The right recurrent laryngeal nerve loops around the right subclavian artery. Because the left recurrent laryngeal nerve has a longer intrathoracic course it is more susceptible to injury (Fig. 1.2).

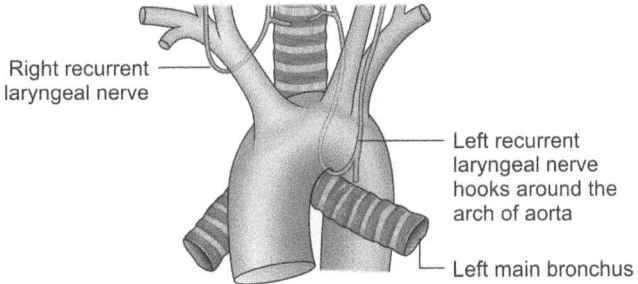

Fig. 1.2: Intrathoracic course of recurrent laryngeal nerve

29. What are the common causes of injury to the recurrent laryngeal nerve?

Noninfectious intrathoracic causes of injury to the recurrent laryngeal nerve include compression of the nerve by lesions in lung and esophageal cancer, mediastinal metastases, lymphoma, sarcoidosis, silicosis etc. Aneurysms of the aortic arch or the dilated left atrium in mitral stenosis can also compress the nerve. Surgical procedures can also damage the nerve.

Tuberculosis is the most common intrathoracic infection causing paralysis of the recurrent laryngeal nerve. This happens as a result of compression of the nerve by mediastinal lymph nodes or entrapment or traction of the nerve by the fibrotic apical tuberculous lesions.

30. What are the important causes of local tenderness of the chest wall?

Chest wall diseases are the cause of chest pain in many patients. Most of the chest wall diseases are associated with local tenderness on palpation. The commonest causes of local tenderness of the chest wall are the following:

- Rib fracture—due to trauma, malignant tumor infiltration, severe bouts of cough etc. The 4th to 10th ribs are most often involved
- Costochondritis—it is a condition characterized by tenderness to palpation of costochondral junctions (usually multiple sites on same side of chest)
- Tietze's syndrome—localized tenderness of costal cartilage of the 2nd rib.
- Tumor infiltration of the chest wall

- Empyema necessitans—occurs in empyema thoracis when the pus in the pleural cavity tracks through and point on the chest wall.

Another important cause of painful dysesthesia in the T4–T12 dermatomes is diabetic truncal neuropathy. It is typically seen in older NIDDM patients.

31. What is the difference between costochondritis and Tietze syndrome?

Costochondritis is a self-limited condition defined as inflammation of costochondral junctions of ribs or chondrosternal joints, usually at multiple levels and lacking swelling or induration. Pain of costochondritis is reproduced by palpation of the affected cartilage segments and may radiate on the chest wall. Costochondritis is often confused with Tietze syndrome, a similar but rarer disorder involving swelling of a single costal cartilage, usually of the second rib (Table 1.6).

Table 1.6: Feature of costochondritis and Tietze syndrome

Feature	Costochondritis	Tietze syndrome
Prevalence	More common	Rare
Age	Older than 40 years	Younger than 40 years
Number of affected sites	More than one	One
Commonly affected costochondral junctions	Second to fifth	Second and third
Local swelling or induration	Absent	Present

32. What is clubbing?

Clubbing is the bulbous uniform swelling of the soft tissue of the terminal phalanx of a digit with subsequent loss of the normal angle between the nail and the nail bed. Clubbing is usually acquired, painless and bilateral. Clubbing usually first develops in the index finger.

Although finger clubbing is relatively innocuous, it is important because of its frequent association with significant underlying diseases. The major conditions that are associated with clubbing are pulmonary diseases (75–80%), cardiovascular abnormalities (10–15%), diseases of the liver and gastrointestinal tract (5–15%) and miscellaneous disorders (5–15%). Finger clubbing may also occur rarely in some people without any evidence of underlying disease. This type of clubbing is called as idiopathic clubbing.

33. What is the mechanism of clubbing?

The pathophysiology behind finger clubbing is not completely understood but the 'platelet hypothesis' offers the most complete explanation. Platelets are derived from megakaryocytes which differentiate from hematopoietic stem cells in the bone marrow. Megakaryocytes and clumps of platelets do not normally reach the arterial circulation. They are released from the bone marrow, but their large size prevents them from passing through the pulmonary capillaries, where they get trapped. There are some conditions where these platelet clumps bypass the pulmonary capillaries and reach the systemic circulation.

These conditions include right to left shunts associated with congenital heart disease or the presence of an infected cardiac valve when these clumps are formed in the peripheral arterial circulation or damage to the pulmonary capillaries in diseases like bronchiectasis and lung abscess. In all such situations, these platelet clumps reach the systemic circulation and gets trapped in the terminal capillaries of the fingers and toes. The platelet derived growth factor (PDGF) released from these trapped platelet clumps cause fibrovascular proliferation. This soft tissue proliferation ultimately produce clubbing. This is the well-accepted humoral or PDGF theory of clubbing.

34. What is floating nail sign in clubbing?

Normally, pressure on the root of the nail bed produces no movement of the nail plate. When there is clubbing, the nail plate is separated from the underlying bone by excess connective tissue and edema. So on applying pressure, the nail moves from side to side and also towards the bone as if it is floating on a cushion. This sign is called as the "Floating nail" sign.

35. What is Lovibond's angle and what is Profile sign?

The angle between the nail-bed and the skin overlying the adjacent part of the distal phlanx is called Lovibond's angle (Fig. 1.3). It is about 180 degrees or less in normal persons. Proliferation of tissues under the nail plate in clubbing causes this angle to increase to more than 180 degrees and this sign is called as the "Profile" sign.

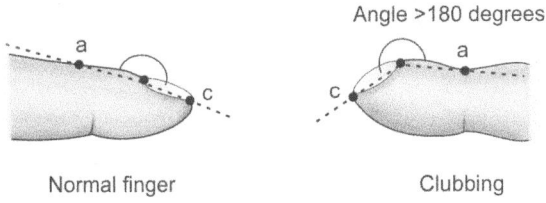

Fig. 1.3: Lovibond's angle

36. What is Schamroth's sign?

Normally when the dorsal surface of terminal phlanges of opposite fingers are opposed there is a diamond shaped window in between them. In clubbing this diamond shaped window is absent and this is called as "Schamroth's" sign (Fig. 1.4).

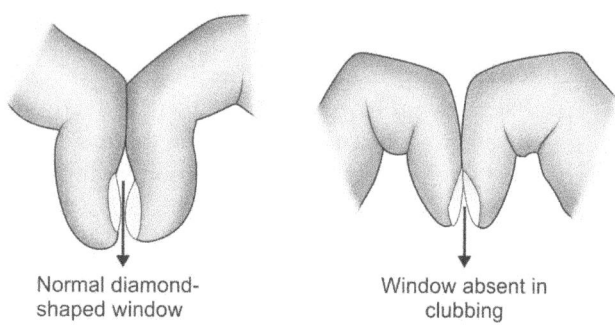

Fig. 1.4: Schamroth's sign

37. What is meant by phalangeal depth ratio?

One objective method to detect early clubbing is the calculation of phalangeal depth ratio. The index finger should be used for measurement as clubbing usually first appears in the index finger (Fig. 1.5).

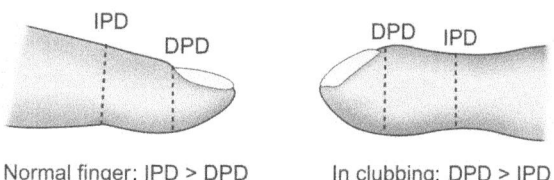

Fig. 1.5: Phalangeal depth ratio

Abbreviations: IPD, interphalangeal depth; DPD, distal phalangeal depth

Phalangeal depth ratio or the DPD / IPD ratio is usually less than 1. A ratio of more than 1 indicates clubbing (DPD is the distal phalengeal depth and IPD is the depth at the distal interphalangeal joint).

38. How is clubbing graded according to severity?

Grade	Description
Grade 1	In this stage, grossly the nail may appear normal. But there is softening of the nail bed and there may be glossiness to the skin adjacent to the nail bed. This results in a spongy sensation on palpation. This is the stage where floating nail sign is present. This sign can be demonstrated using the index fingers of the examiner, after fixing the patient's clubbed finger with the thumbs of the examiner's hands as shown below. Pressing the base of finger to look for fluctuation of nail bed
Grade 2	Curvature of the nail bed increases leading to obliteration of the diamond shaped space created by opposing the dorsal surface of the terminal phalanx of identical fingers from either hand (i.e. positive Schamroth's sign). Lovibond's angle is also lost. Loss of Lovibond's angle

Contd...

Contd...

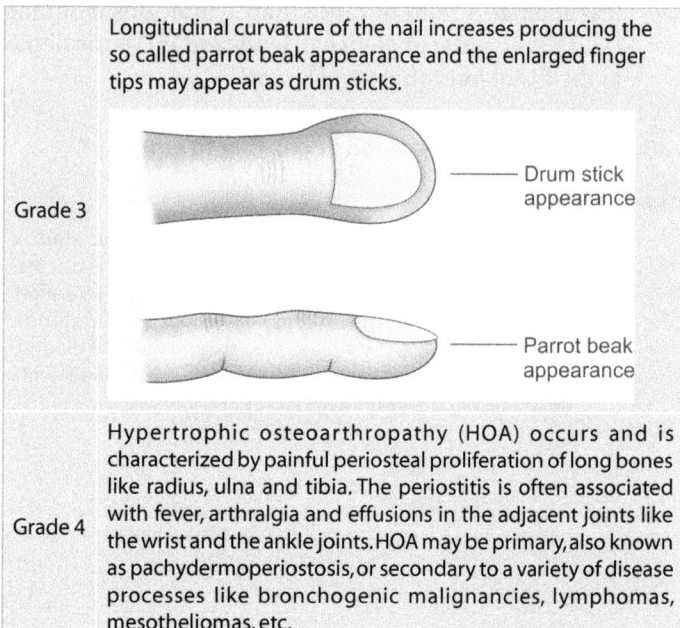

Grade 3	Longitudinal curvature of the nail increases producing the so called parrot beak appearance and the enlarged finger tips may appear as drum sticks.
Grade 4	Hypertrophic osteoarthropathy (HOA) occurs and is characterized by painful periosteal proliferation of long bones like radius, ulna and tibia. The periostitis is often associated with fever, arthralgia and effusions in the adjacent joints like the wrist and the ankle joints. HOA may be primary, also known as pachydermoperiostosis, or secondary to a variety of disease processes like bronchogenic malignancies, lymphomas, mesotheliomas, etc.

39. What is pseudoclubbing?

Pseudoclubbing is due to subperiosteal bone resorption of terminal phlanges without soft tissue proliferation. So, the fundamental angle between the nail bed and the terminal phlanx is not altered. It may be seen in persons with increased nail curvature, chronic paronychiae, abscesses of the terminal pulp space, etc.

40. What are the common causes of clubbing?

The mnemonic "CCLLUBBIING" is a reminder of the common causes for clubbing and they are the following (Box 1.4):

> **Box 1.4:** Causes of clubbing
>
> - **C**yanotic congenital heart diseases and **C**ystic fibrosis
> - **L**ung cancer (usually non-small cell types) and **L**ung abscess
> - **U**lcerative colitis and Crohn's disease
> - **B**ronchiectasis
> - **B**iliary cirrhosis
> - **I**nfective endocarditis and **I**nterstitial lung disease
> - **N**eurogenic diaphragmatic tumors
> - **G**rave's disease (referred to as thyroid acropachy)

Unilateral upper extremity clubbing may occur in conditions like anomalies of the aortic arch, aortic or subclavian artery aneurysm, pancoast tumor, hemiplegia, etc. Isolated clubbing of toes without involvement of fingers is seen in coarctation of aorta. Unidigital clubbing can occur in trauma.

41. What is cyanosis and what is the role of arterial blood gas analysis in diagnosing hypoxemia in a person with cyanosis?

The bluish discoloration of the skin and mucous membranes due to the increased quantity of deoxyhemoglobin (atleast 5 g/dL) or hemoglobin derivatives like methemoglobin or sulfhemoglobin in the subpapillary capillaries is defined as cyanosis. It is usually seen on the tongue (most sensitive area), lips, ears, malar eminences and the nail beds.

Cyanosis as a tool for detecting arterial hypoxemia is neither sensitive nor specific. Severe hypoxemia may be present at times when cyanosis is not detectable either because of observer insensitivity or confounding factors such as heavy melanin pigmentation or severe anemia (Hb less than 5 g/dL) in the patient. So, arterial blood gas analysis is very important in confirming hypoxemia.

42. What is the difference between central and peripheral cyanosis?

Central cyanosis occurs when the oxygenation of arterial blood in the lungs is reduced or when excessive amount of an abnormal hemoglobin derivative like methemoglobin is present in the blood. Since the defect is in the central mechanism, cyanosis can be seen simultaneously in the mucous membranes as well as on the skin of the peripheral parts of the body.

Peripheral cyanosis is due to the abnormal excessive extraction of oxygen from the normally saturated arterial blood in the peripheral circulation. This usually results from diminished or sluggish peripheral blood flow due to vasoconstriction (e.g. exposure to cold, peripheral vascular disease, etc.). Hence cyanosis can be seen only on the skin of the affected part of the body where there is vasoconstriction (Table 1.7).

Table 1.7: Difference between central and peripheral cyanosis

Central cyanosis	Peripheral cyanosis
• Involves skin and mucous membranes	• Only skin is involved
• Nail beds are deep blue	• Nail beds are pale
• Skin is warm	• Skin is cold and clammy
• May improve with oxygen therapy	• May improve by applying warmth

Cyanosis occurring in conditions like cardiogenic shock is due to both the above mechanisms of production of cyanosis, and this type of cyanosis is referred to as mixed cyanosis (Fig. 1.6).

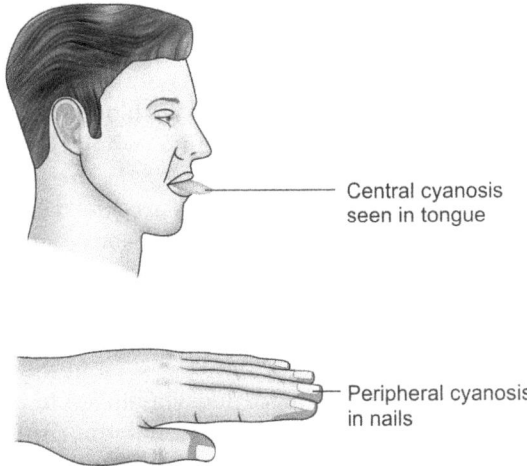

Fig. 1.6: Central versus peripheral cyanosis

43. Which are the pigments and drugs causing bluish discolouration of skin?

Ingestion of substances containing gold or silver can cause bluish discoloration of the skin that is more prominent in the sun exposed areas. The bluish skin color caused by deposition of hemosiderin is more apparent in areas with less melanotic pigment. Oxidation products of the drug chlorpromazine, when deposited in the skin, can result in a bluish color. Prolonged use of amiodarone, can cause lipofuscin deposition in the skin which produces a bluish discoloration.

44. What is the mechanism of production of ruddy cyanosis?

Ruddy cyanosis is a type of deep cyanosis with a reddish blue tinge seen in conditions were there is polycythemia with or without hypoxia. A minimum of about 5 g/dL of deoxyhemoglobin should be there for cyanosis to become clinically apparent. The amount of deoxyhemoglobin in blood is directly proportional to the amount of total hemoglobin in the blood.

Therefore, in severe anemia, when the quantity of hemoglobin is less than 5 g/dL, the amount of deoxyhemoglobin that can be produced is also less than 5 g/dL. So, even in the presence of hypoxia, cyanosis is not demonstrable in severe anemia. Conversely, in chronic hypoxic diseases like COPD, there is secondary polycythemia with increased amount of total hemoglobin. So, even in the absence of hypoxia, the amount of deoxyhemoglobin produced in these individuals is high. Hence the combination of polycythemia and hypoxia in COPD patients is responsible for a peculiar type of cyanosis with a slight reddish tinge called as the ruddy cyanosis.

45. What is facial plethora?

Facial plethora is a weather-beaten facial appearance seen in polycythemia, resulting from a combination of excessive redness (due to the very high concentration of hemoglobin) and cyanosis. It is important to remember that in primary polycythemia (also called as polycythemia vera), there may be enough deoxyhemoglobin to produce cyanosis even in the absence of hypoxia. This is attributed to the increased red cell mass in this condition.

46. What is differential cyanosis?

Differential cyanosis is seen in patent ductus arteriosus (PDA) with reversal of the left to right shunt (Fig. 1.7). Here deoxygenated blood flows from the pulmonary artery to the aorta (through the ductus) distal to the origin of the carotid and subclavian arteries. Hence, the feet are cyanosed but the hands are pink (right hand is pinker than left).

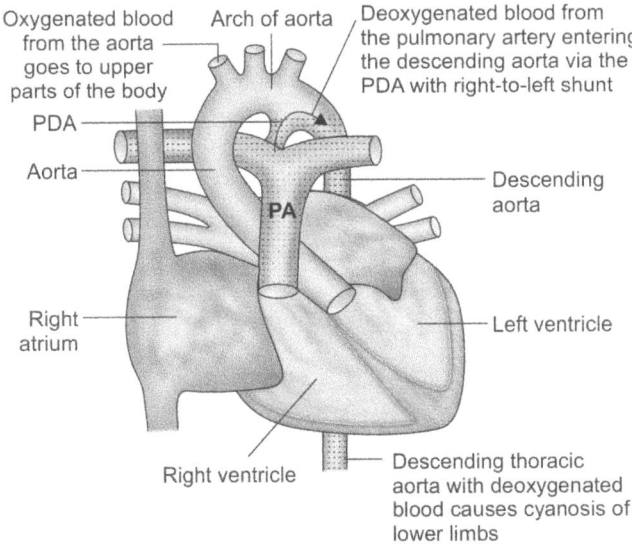

Fig. 1.7: Mechanism of differential cyanosis

Reversed differential cyanosis is a rare but important physical sign. In this condition, the toes are pink and the hands are blue. It is seen in complete transposition of great arteries associated with pulmonary hypertension and PDA.

47. How will you distinguish neck vein distension due to cor pulmonale from that of superior venacaval syndrome?

Cor pulmonale is defined as enlargement (dilatation and/or hypertrophy) of the right ventricle due to increased right ventricular afterload secondary to abnormalities of the chest wall, lungs, pulmonary ventilation or pulmonary circulation. Superior vena cava syndrome is the result of obstruction of the superior vena cava.

Facial puffiness, headache, conjunctival suffusion and neck vein distension can occur in both entities. However, in superior vena cava syndrome there is nonpulsatile neck vein distension with negative hepatojugular reflex, and there is prominent superficial vascularity of neck and upper chest. In corpulmonale there is pulsatile neck vein distension with positive hepatojugular reflex (Table 1.8).

Table 1.8: Difference between cor pulmonale and superior vena cava obstruction

Cor pulmonale	Superior vena cava obstruction
Distended neck veins are pulsatile	Distended neck veins are non-pulsatile
Positive hepatojugular reflex	Negative hepatojugular reflex

48. What is asterixis or "flapping" tremor?

Asterixis, which may superficially resemble a tremor, is actually an intermittent inhibition of muscle contraction that leads to repetitive partial flexion of the wrists during attempted sustained wrist extension. It can be elicited by asking the person to hyperextend his arms at the elbow and wrist with the fingers spread apart. Asterixis was first described in hepatic encephalopathy (Box 1.5).

Box 1.5: Causes of asterixis

- Hepatic encephalopathy
- Uremia
- Hypokalemia
- Hypomagnesemia
- Carbon dioxide narcosis
- Dialysis dementia

49. What is the influence of respiration on the blood pressure and heart rate?

Under normal conditions, the arterial blood pressure fluctuates throughout the respiratory cycle. During inspiration there is a fall in the left ventricular stroke volume due to a combination of reversed Bernheim effect, increased pooling of blood in the lungs and negative intrathoracic pressure. This is reflected as a fall in the systolic blood pressure. The converse is true for expiration.

During quiet respiration, the variations in the intrathoracic pressures are small and so the changes in the blood pressure are also minor. The accepted upper limit for the fall in systolic blood pressure with inspiration is 10 mm Hg. An exaggerated fall in the systolic blood pressure (>10 mm Hg) during inspiration is referred to as pulsus paradoxus.

Normally, there should be an increase in the heart rate during inspiration. This is a physiological response and it is more accentuated in children. This is referred to as sinus arrhythmia (Fig. 1.8). Absence of this normal variation in heart rate with breathing is a feature of autonomic neuropathy.

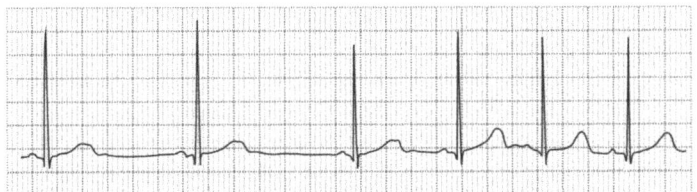

Fig. 1.8: Marked sinus arrhythmia

Sinus arrhythmia can be easily distinguished from atrial extrasystoles, because in sinus arrhythmia, all the P waves have the same morphology.

50. What is the mechanism of pulsus paradoxus in severe bronchial asthma?

Pulsus paradoxus is one of the ominous signs in acute exacerbation of bronchial asthma and this is the most common extracardiac cause of this physical sign. The main mechanisms behind the genesis of pulsus paradoxus in bronchial asthma are the following:
- The unusually great fluctuations in the intrathoracic pressures that are transmitted to the aorta
- Hyperinflation of the chest due to air trapping.

The clinical method of assessment of this pulse is by measurement of the systolic blood pressure using sphygmomanometer.

51. Which are the important respiratory diseases that can cause lymphadenopathy?

The three diseases commonly causing lymphadenopathy are tuberculosis, bronchogenic malignancy and sarcoidosis. Tuberculous lymphadenitis (scrofula) is the most common form of extrapulmonary tuberculosis. It is more common in children and young adults than in older persons. Cervical lymph nodes are affected most commonly and they are usually matted, painless and nontender. Occasionally, the patients fail to show any constitutional features such as fever or night sweats. However, the tuberculin test is usually strongly positive. "Collar-stud" abscesses and sinus formation may occur later in untreated cases. It should be remembered that during antituberculous therapy, an immune response to killed mycobacteria may initially cause new nodes to appear. Lymph node excision is indicated only for diagnostic purpose.

Supraclavicular, scalene and axillary lymphnodes may be involved in bronchogenic malignancy. Axillary lymph nodes are involved in chest wall and pleural lesions. The right supraclavicular lymph node is involved in lesions of the right lung and left lower lobe. The left supraclavicular lymph node (Virchow's node) is involved in lesions of the left upper lobe (a palpable Virchow's node is referred to as Troisier's sign). The scalene lymph node lies on the scalenus anticus muscle (Fig. 1.9).

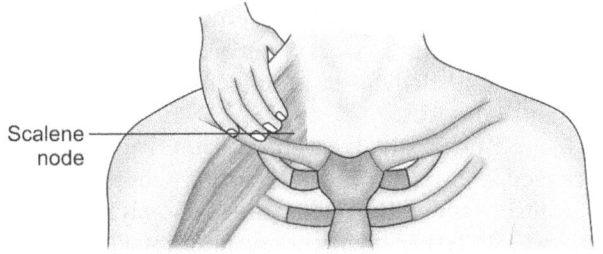

Fig. 1.9: Palpation of the scalene lymph node behind the clavicle

Sarcoidosis is a multisystem granulomatous disorder. The mediastinal and superficial lymph glands, lungs, liver, spleen, skin, eyes, parotid glands and phalangeal bones are the most frequently affected tissues. The characteristic histological feature is a noncaseating epithelioid granuloma. Disturbances in calcium metabolism may lead to hypercalcemia. Sarcoidosis may cause bilateral hilar lymphadenopathy (70-90%) and this type of sarcoidosis with hilar adenopathy, erythema nodosum and joint symptoms is referred to as the Lofgren's syndrome.

52. What do you know about Kikuchi's disease?

Kikuchi's disease, also called Kikuchi-Fujimoto disease or Kikuchi's histiocytic necrotizing lymphadenitis, is a rare, benign condition of unknown cause usually characterized by cervical lymphadenopathy and low grade fever. Systemic symptoms may accompany fever and lymphadenopathy. Systemic symptoms include night sweats, nausea, vomiting, weight loss etc. Hence, this diaease may cause diagnostic confusion with tuberculosis. Most patients are younger than 40 years of age. While the pathogenesis of Kikuchi's disease is unknown, the clinical presentation, course, and histologic changes suggest an immune response of T cells and histiocytes to an infectious agent, such as Epstein-Barr virus.

Lymph node involvement is usually cervical and localized, although some patients have more extensive node involvement. The nodes are usually only moderately enlarged (1-2 cm in diameter) but occasionally are much larger. They are typically firm, smooth, discrete and mobile. The nodal enlargement is often associated with dull or acute pain.

The majority of patients with Kikuchi's disease have a normal blood count but erythrocyte sendimentation rate (ESR) is usually high. The diagnosis of Kikuchi's disease is made by lymph node biopsy. Biopsy should be performed, despite the self-limited nature of this syndrome, in order to exclude more serious conditions requiring aggressive therapy such as tuberculosis or lymphoma. No effective treatment has been established for Kikuchi's disease. Signs and symptoms usually resolve within one to four months. Patients with severe or persisting symptoms have been treated with glucocorticoids with apparent benefit.

53. Which are the drugs causing lymphadenopathy?

A number of medications may cause serum sickness that is characterized by fever, arthralgias, rash and generalized lymphadenopathy. They include the following (Box 1.6).

Box 1.6: Drugs causing lymphadenopathy

- Phenytoin
- Sulfonamides
- Carbamazepine
- Atenolol
- Pencillin
- Cephalosporins
- Quinidine
- Captopril

It is to be remembered that, phenytoin can cause generalized lymphadenopathy in the absence of a serum sickness reaction.

54. What is Waldeyer's ring?

The Waldeyer's ring is constituted by a circular chain of lymphoid tissues. The internal Waldeyer's ring is formed by adenoids, palatine tonsils, tubal tonsils and the lingual tonsil. The external Waldeyer's ring is another chain formed by the occipital, post- and preauricular, jugular, submandibular and submental groups of lymph nodes. Waldeyer's ring adenopathy occurs in case of local diseases or it may be a part of generalized lymphadenopathy in conditions like lymphoma (Fig. 1.10).

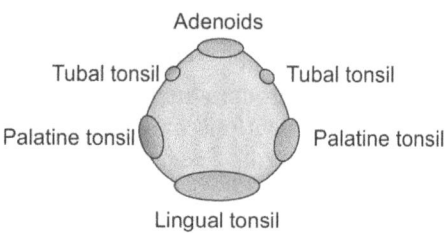

Fig. 1.10: Internal ring

55. What are the immunological manifestations seen in primary tuberculosis?

The common immunological phenomenon seen in primary pulmonary tuberculosis include erythema nodosum and phlyctenular conjunctivitis. Erythema nodosum consists of bluish red, tender subcutaneous nodules most commonly seen on the shins (sometimes on the thighs). The lesions represent a delayed hypersensitivity reaction to antigens associated with various infectious agents like the tubercle bacilli. It is also seen in conditions like sarcoidosis, streptococcal infections and in some drug reactions.

Phlyctenular conjunctivitis consists of hard, red, raised 1–3 mm nodules accompanied by a zone of hyperemia located near the limbus on the bulbar conjunctiva of the eye.

56. What do you know about tuberculous rheumatism?

Tuberculous rheumatism or Poncet's disease is a rare "reactive" acute symmetrical polyarthritis involving large and small joints. It is associated with active pulmonary or extrapulmonary tuberculosis. There is no evidence of active tuberculous infection of the involved joints. Pathogenesis is unclear, although evidence suggests an immune-mediated phenomenon. HIV coinfection may be a risk factor. The arthritis resolves within a few weeks of initiation of antituberculosis therapy with no residual joint destruction.

57. What physical examination findings in the abdomen would you look for while examining a patient with lung disease?

Some important signs that have to be specifically looked for while examining the abdomen of a patient with lung disease are the following:

- Abdominal wall and inguinal hernias due to chronic cough in COPD
- Firm tender smooth hepatomegaly and ascites—as a result of chronic liver congestion (cardiac cirrhosis) due to right heart failure in cor pulmonale
- Hard irregular nontender hepatomegaly—metastasis from lung malignancy
- Ptosed or pushed down liver—seen in emphysema (liver span is normal)
- Splenomegaly—due to amyloidosis in chronic suppurative diseases like bronchiectasis, tuberculosis, etc.

58. Which are the muscles involved in the act of respiration?

In normal respiration, inspiration is an active movement aided mainly by the diaphragm and the external intercostal muscles. Transverse thoracic diameter is increased by fixing the first rib and raising the other ribs to it (bucket handle movement). This is done by the intercostal muscles. Anteroposterior diameter is increased by moving up the body of sternum (pump handle movement). Both these movements cause expansion of the thoracic cavity, leading to an increase in the intrathoracic negative pressure. This results in the expansion of the lung. Expiration is normally a passive movement depending on the elastical recoil of the lung and the chest wall (Fig. 1.11).

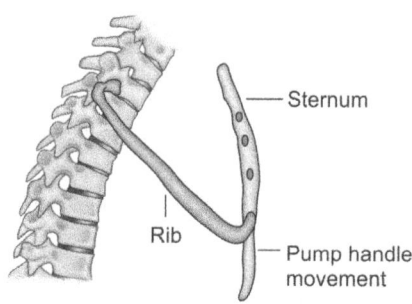

Fig. 1.11: Pump handle movement elevating the sternum

However, in disease states, accessory muscles come into action. The main accessory muscles of inspiration are the scalene, serratus anterior, pectoralis minor and sternocleidomastoid muscles. The main accessory muscles of expiration are the muscles of the anterior abdominal wall, internal intercostal muscles and the lattisimus dorsi.

59. What is the clinical significance of hyperpnea?

The normal respiratory rate in an adult is 16 to 18 per minute. If the rate is more than 24 per minute, then it is referred to as tachypnea. Hyperpnea, on the other hand, is the term used when the depth of breathing is markedly increased. When associated with rapid breaths, hyperpnea seems to be a reliable sign of metabolic acidosis and this deep and rapid breathing is called as the Kussmaul's breathing. The deep breaths help to washout carbon dioxide from the body, creating respiratory alkalosis, as a compensation to the metabolic acidosis.

60. What is the physiological basis of Cheyne-Stokes respiration?

Cheyne-Stokes respiration is an abnormal type of respiration where periods of rapid breathing alternate with periods of apnea (apnea means pause of breathing for 10 seconds). During the apnea phase there is carbon dioxide retention. This stimulates the respiratory center which in turn causes rapid breathing. This rapid breathing causes carbon dioxide washout leading to depression of the respiratory center. This in turn leads to the phase of apnea and the same cycle again repeats. Common causes of Cheyne-Stokes respiration include heart failure, uremia, drug induced respiratory depression and extensive cerebral damage (Fig. 1.12).

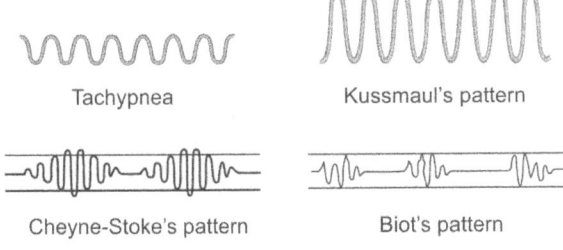

Fig. 1.12: Patterns of respiration

Another type of periodic breathing is the Biot's respiration or cluster breathing which consists of clusters of irregular breaths that alternate with periods of apnea. But this type of breathing does not have the crescendo-decrescendo pattern seen with the Cheyne-Stoke's respiration. Biot's respiration can occur in brainstem lesions.

61. What is Ondine's curse?

Congenital central hypoventilation syndrome or CCHS, is a disorder of the central nervous system where the automatic control of breathing is absent or impaired. In this condition, the response to hypoxia or hypercapnia is typically sluggish during awake hours and absent, to varying degrees, during sleep. CCHS should be considered in children with episodic or sustained hypoventilation without obvious cardiopulmonary or neuromuscular disease. Ondine's or Undine's curse is a rare severe form of CCHS characterized by respiratory arrest during sleep.

62. What is hyperventilation syndrome?

Hyperventilation syndrome or HVS is a condition in which minute ventilation exceeds metabolic demands. A better term for this syndrome is behavioral breathlessness or psychogenic dyspnea, with hyperventilation seen as a consequence rather than a cause of the condition. The peak incidence is between the ages of 15 and 55 years. Approximately 50% of patients with panic disorder and 60% of patients with agoraphobia manifest hyperventilation as a symptom. Many persons who are affected, appear to have an abnormal respiratory response to stress and other chemical and emotional triggers, which results in excess minute ventilation.

In most patients with HVS, the mechanics of breathing is disordered in a characteristic way. When stressed, these patients rely on thoracic breathing rather than diaphragmatic breathing, resulting in a hyperexpanded chest and high residual lung volume. Because of the high residual volume, they are unable to take a normal tidal volume with the next breath and consequently experience dyspnea. Proprioceptors in the lung and chest wall signal the brain with a "suffocation alarm" that triggers the release of excitatory neurotransmitters that are responsible for many of the symptoms such as palpitations, tremor, anxiety and diaphoresis.

63. What is the reason for carpopedal spasm in hyperventilation syndrome?

Hyperventilation syndrome results in respiratory alkalosis. Alkalosis promotes the binding of calcium to albumin and can reduce the fraction of ionized calcium in the blood (even in the presence of normal total calcium level). The clinical manifestation of hypocalcemia is associated with overexcitabilty of sensory and motor neurons. This causes twitching of the ipsilateral facial muscles, upon stimulation of the facial nerve by tapping on the face at a point just anterior to the ear (i.e. positive Chvostek's sign) and also flexion of the wrist and metacarpophalangeal joints, hyperextension of the fingers and flexion of the thumb on to the palm, during measurement of systolic blood pressure using a sphygmomanometer cuff (i.e. positive Trousseau's sign) (Fig. 1.13).

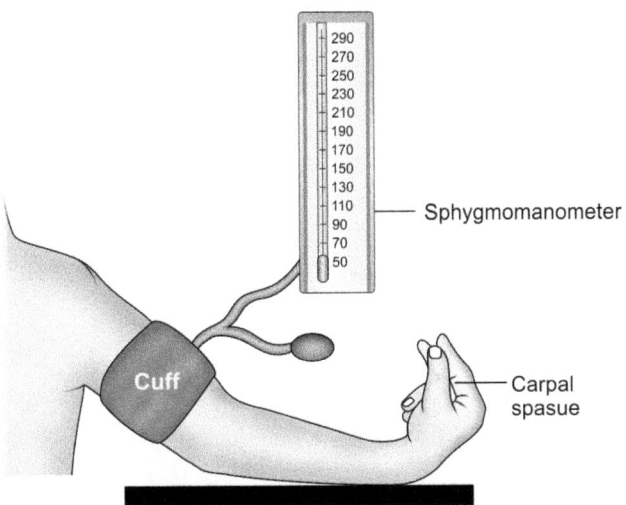

Fig. 1.13: Elicitation of Trousseau's sign

64. What is meant by sighing respiration?

Sighing pattern of respiration is usually seen in psychogenic dyspnea. It is characterized by an occasional deep and audible sigh that punctuates an otherwise regular respiratory pattern. In those with psychogenic dyspnea, these sighs occur too frequently. Sometimes sighs also occur in normal regular respiration (Fig. 1.14).

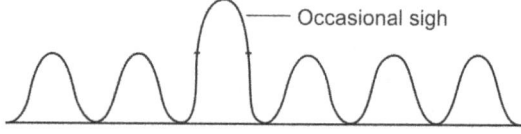

Fig. 1.14: Sighing pattern of respiration

Chapter 2

Inspection and Palpation of the Chest Wall

1. **What do you know about the pectus deformities of the chest wall?**

   Pectus deformities are the most common congenital chest wall deformities and are better known as pigeon chest and funnel chest. In case of pectus excavatum (i.e. funnel chest) the sternum is depressed in a concave shape and in pectus carinatum (i.e. pigeon chest) the sternum is protruded in a convex shape. Both these deformities are more common in males.

   The coexistence of pectus excavatum with other musculoskeletal disorders, such as Marfan syndrome, suggests that an abnormality of connective tissue may be involved in the genesis of this condition. In addition, 40% of patients with pectus excavatum have a familial history, suggesting a possible genetic predisposition. Pectus carinatum is frequently caused by severe asthma during childhood. Very occasionally, this deformity can be produced by rickets or be idiopathic.

2. **What are the cardiovascular findings expected in a person with pectus excavatum?**

   Pectus excavatum or funnel chest is an exaggeration of normal depression seen at end of the sternum. It is commonly seen in Marfan syndrome and Straight back syndrome and is usually asymptomatic. But when there is marked degree of depression of the sternum, the heart may be compressed and the cardiac apex is shifted to left. Also, the second heart sound may be widely split and there may be a mid-systolic murmur along the left sternal border.

3. What is the peculiarity of barrel-shaped chest?

In normal adults, the anteroposterior diameter of the thorax is shorter than the transverse diameter, in a ratio of **5:7** and the chest is elliptical in cross-section. In elderly and in those with diseases like chronic obstructive airway disease, the anteroposterior diameter is more than or equal to the transverse diameter, thereby making the chest cylindrical or barrel shaped in cross-section (Fig. 2.1A).

In barrel-shaped chest, the ribs are horizontal (subcostal angle >90) and the diaphragm is pushed to a more downward flat position so as to accommodate the hyperinflated lungs. Barrel-shaped architecture is an physiological adaptation in COPD patients because this shape would expand the thoracic cavity and lift the lung away from the collapsing airways. This helps to reduce the external forces compressing the airway lumen (Fig. 2.1B).

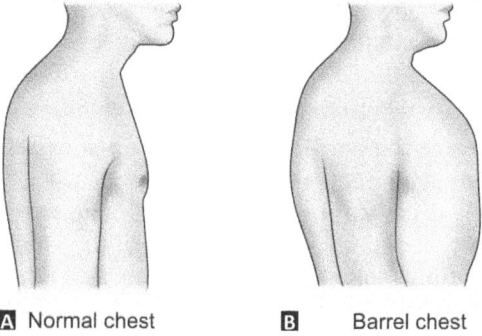

A Normal chest B Barrel chest

Figs 2.1A and B: Comparison of normal and barrel-shaped chest

4. What is the effect of barrel-shaped chest on the efficiency of respiration?

Normally during inspiration the ribs move outward (bucket handle movement) and upward (pump handle movement) and the diaphragm move downwards leading to the expansion of the thorax. This expansion of the thoracic cage increases the intrathoracic negative pressure and this results in air being sucked into the lungs, thereby causing expansion of the lungs.

In those with barrel chest, because of the horizontal ribs and low lying flat diaphragm, only the upward movement of ribs occur effectively and this cannot sufficiently expand the thoracic cage and generate the negative pressure needed to suck in air into the lungs. Hence, the accessory muscles of respiration come into action and so the work of breathing is more in barrel shaped chest but the efficiency of respiration is less. This causes severe physical exhaustion of the patient and he may develop "pulmonary cachexia".

5. How will you assess the severity of kyphosis and what is its significance?

Kyphosis or " humpback " is the forward bending of the vertebral column and scoliosis is the lateral bending of the vertebral column. In normal persons there is a mild thoracic kyphosis. An important cause of hyperkyphosis in elderly is osteoporotic fractures of the vertebrae.

Severity of kyphosis is objectively assessed by calculating the Cobb's angle from X-rays of the spine (lateral view). An angle of more than 45 degrees is considered as pathological kyphosis (Fig. 2.2).

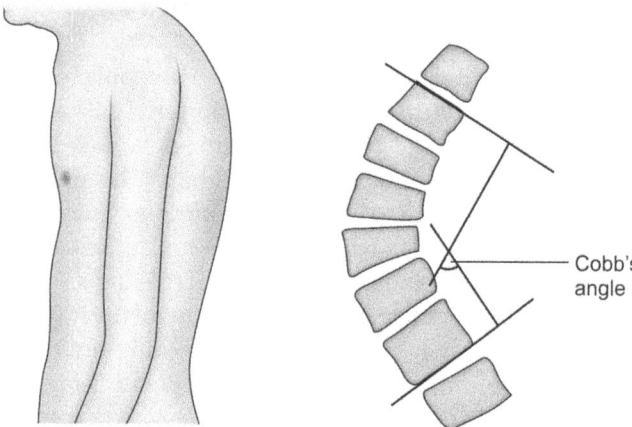

Fig. 2.2: Kyphosis and method of calculating the Cobb's angle

The distortion of the chest wall leads to reduction in the lung volume and increases the stiffness of the chest wall, thereby causing a restrictive ventilatory defect and increase the work of breathing. Patients with severe deformity may develop type II respiratory failure, pulmonary hypertension and right ventricular failure.

6. How will you differentiate between scoliosis due to lung pathology from compensatory scoliosis due to short leg on one side?

Compensatory scoliosis disappears when the person sits down or bends forward. In scoliosis due to lung pathology the convexity of the spine is towards the opposite side of the lung lesion and the scoliosis persists even when the person sits down or bends forward.

7. What are the factors that influence the type of breathing?

The type of breathing depends on the sex and age of the person. In women, the respiratory movements mainly involves the upper part of the thorax and this type of respiration is called as thoracoabdominal respiration. In men and children, the respiratory movements are mainly abdominal and this type of respiration is called as the abdominothoracic respiration.

8. What is meant by "prefixed trachea"?

Normally, lesions like pleural effusion and pneumothorax causes the trachea to be shifted to the opposite side of the lesion, whereas fibrosis and collapse causes tracheal shift towards the same side of the lesion. However, if the trachea is already displaced and fixed by a past illness of the lung (e.g. old tuberculosis with resultant fibrosis), then we may not get the tracheal shift that is expected with the present lung pathology. In such situations, the trachea is said to be "prefixed".

9. What is the mechanism behind positive Trail's sign?

Undue prominence of the clavicular head of sternocleidomastoid muscle on the same side to which the trachea is displaced is called as positive Trail's sign. When the trachea is shifted to one side, the pretracheal fascia which encloses the sternocleidomastoid muscle on the same side relaxes. This makes the clavicular head of the muscle more prominent on that side.

10. What are the physical signs elicited during inspection of a COPD patient?

The important physical signs that can be elicited in patients with chronic airway obstruction are the following:

- Reduction in the length of trachea palpable above the sternal notch (i.e. less than 3 finger breadths)
- Tracheal descent with inspiration (Campbell's sign)
- Use of the accessory muscles of respiration
- Pursed lip breathing (helps to prevent expiratory airway collapse)

- Excavation of the suprasternal and supraclavicular fossae during inspiration
- Jugular venous filling during expiration
- Loss of bucket-handle (outward) movement of the upper ribs
- Paradoxical inward movement of the lower ribs during inspiration results in a decrease in the costal angle (Hoover's sign)
- Sits in a leaning forward position supporting the hands on their knees. This is called as the tripod position
- Edema due to cor pulmonale or CO_2 retention. CO_2 dilates the afferent renal arterioles more than the efferents. This leads to fluid retention by the kidneys (*Ref: Bedside Cardiology, Jules Constant*).

11. What is tracheal tug?

Tracheal tug or Oliver's sign is an abnormal downward movement of the trachea during systole that indicates either a dilatation or aneurysm of the aortic arch. It is elicited by gently grasping the cricoid cartilage and applying upward pressure while the patient stands with his chin extended upward. A downward tug or pull of the trachea may be felt if aneurysm is present.

12. What are the clinical signs of volume loss of a hemithorax observed on the chest wall?

Volume loss of a hemithorax can be caused by either fibrosis or collapse of the lung tissue. Clinical signs of volume loss include the following:

- Shift of trachea towards the side of volume loss
- Shift of cardiac apical impulse towards the side of volume loss

- Hollowing of supraclavicular, infraclavicular and intercoastal spaces on the side of volume loss
- Skeletal changes like crowding of ribs, drooping of shoulder, kyphosis, scoliosis, etc. on the side of volume loss

The presence of skeletal changes in a patient is in favor of fibrosis as the etiology of the volume loss. The most common causes of upper lobe fibrosis are pulmonary tuberculosis, exposure to radiotherapy and rheumatoid arthritis. The most common causes of lower lobe fibrosis are bronchiectasis, asbestosis and fibrosing alveolitis. Isolated shift of the trachea without the shift of cardiac apex indicates upper lobe fibrosis, whereas combined shift of both the trachea and the cardiac apex indicates widespread fibrosis involving both the upper and lower lobes.

13. What is fibrothorax?

Fibrothorax results from fibrosis of the visceral pleura surrounding the lung, and is clinically manifested by decreased respiratory excursion and a restrictive pulmonary physiology.

There are two distinct mechanisms that can lead to the formation of fibrothorax. Most often, fibrothorax develops as a result of pleural inflammation in patients with pleural effusion. This commonly occurs in incompletely evacuated hemothorax, tuberculous effusion or chronic empyema. Fibrothorax can also result from pulmonary parenchymal disease, and can be seen in patients with inadequately treated pulmonary tuberculosis, bronchiectasis or lung abscess. Fibrinous changes can occur to the pleural plaques in asbestosis resulting in fibrothorax.

14. What are the most common causes for collapse (atelectasis) of lung lobes?

Collapse is defined as diminished volume affecting all or part of a lung. Based on the mechanism producing the collapse or atelectasis, there are actually two main types of lung collapse.

The first variant is the obstructive or active collapse and it is the most common type of lung collapse. The term "collapse" usually means obstructive collapse. Obstructive collapse results from reabsorption of gas from the alveoli when the communication between the alveoli and the trachea is obstructed by a foreign body, tumor or mucus plug. The obstruction can occur at the level of the larger bronchus (lobar collapse) or smaller bronchus (segmental collapse).

One of the commonest cause of obstructive collapse of large bronchi is mediastinal lymphadenopahty. The common causes of mediastinal lymphadenopathy are the following (Box 2.1):

Box 2.1: Causes of mediastinal lymphadenopathy

- Secondaries from bronchogenic malignancy
- Tuberculosis
- Lymphoma
- Sarcoidosis

The second type of lung collapse is the non-obstructive collapse which is caused by any one of the following mechanisms.

- Loss of contact between the parietal and visceral pleurae as in pleural effusion or pneumothorax. This is referred to as passive collapse.

- Compression by large space occupying lesions of the thorax (e.g. a massive pleural effusion or a large intrathoracic neoplasm which compresses the adjacent lung tissue and force the air out of the alveoli). This is referred to as compression collapse.
- Loss of surfactant as in ARDS.
- Replacement of parenchymal tissue by scarring or infiltrative disease.

So "passive collapse" and "compression collapse" are actually two subtypes of nonobstructive lung collapse.

15. What are the differences between obstructive collapse and compression collapse?

The classic signs of "collapse" are elicited in a case of obstructive collapse of a lung lobe and they include the following (Fig. 2.3):

- Shift of trachea and cardiac apex towards the same side of collapse
- Decreased lung expansion on the side of collapse
- Dull percussion note on the side of collapse
- Absent breath sounds on the side of collapse since there is no airflow through the obstructed bronchus.

In case of compression collapse, the clinical findings are dominated by the physical signs of the massive thoracic lesion (like large pleural effusion or thoracic tumor) which is producing the compression. So, the trachea and cardiac apex are shifted to the opposite side of compression collapse.

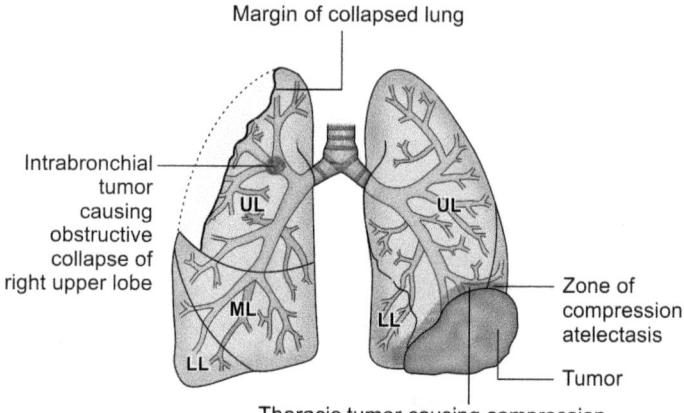

Fig. 2.3: Obstructive versus compression collapse

In case of a large pleural effusion producing compression collapse, some signs like tubular bronchial breath sounds and increased vocal resonance (in the form of egophony) may be elicited just above the upper level of the effusion on the posterolateral chest wall, at the site of compression collapse. This is because the compressed airless lung tissue in that area may transmit the tubular breath sounds from a nearby patent large bronchus directly to the chest wall without filteration. This entity is sometimes referred to as "collapse with patent bronchus".

16. What is meant by "abdominal paradox" and how is it assessed clinically?

Abdominal paradox is defined as the indrawing of the abdominal wall when the rib cage expand outwards during lung inflation. It is due to the abdominal pressure becoming negative during inspiration, and is a sign of major diaphragmatic palsy. This can be clinically assessed by placing one hand of the examiner on the anterior chest wall of the patient and the other hand over the epigastrium of the patient. Normally both the hands of the examiner are lifted during inspiration. But in diaphragmatic palsy, when the hand on the chest wall moves outwards, the other hand on the epigastrium moves inward. Unilateral diaphragmatic palsy can be demonstrated by eliciting the Litten's sign, which shows unilateral absence or diminished abdominal movement.

17. How can you clinically diagnose a mass lesion in the lung?

The only direct clinical evidence of a mass lesion in the lung is a visible or palpable swelling on the chest wall as occurs only in the case of a large lesion. All other evidences are indirect signs that support the final etiological diagnosis as a possible mass lesion. These indirect evidences vary depending on whether the mass lesion is centrally or peripherally located. Some indirect clinical signs like clubbing and lymphadenopathy are common to both central and peripheral neoplasms.

The common centrally placed neoplasms are squamous cell tumors and small cell tumors (Fig. 2.4). They usually present with the following features:
- Hoarseness of voice and bovine cough (non-explosive cough)—due to recurrent laryngeal nerve infiltration.
- Horner's syndrome—due to sympathetic chain infiltration.
- Diaphragmatic palsy—due to phrenic nerve infiltration.
- Superior vena cava syndrome—due to obstruction of the superior vena cava.
- Paraneoplastic syndromes—common with small cell lung cancer.

- Collapse of the lung lobes—due to bronchial obstruction
- Recurrent or nonresolving pneumonia—due to bronchial obstruction.

The common peripherally located neoplasms are adenocarcinoma and large cell carcinoma (Fig. 2.5). Adenocarcimoma is the most common type of bronchogenic malignancy in females, in non smokers and in young persons (less than 40 years). The peripheral neoplasms usually present with the following features:

- Chest pain—due to malignant pleural effusion and rib erosions
- Bronchorrhea—due to profuse thin mucoid sputum production (more than 100 mL/day) and is seen in broncholoalveolar cell variant of adenocarcinoma.
- Lobular pneumonic consolidation
- Pleural effusion.

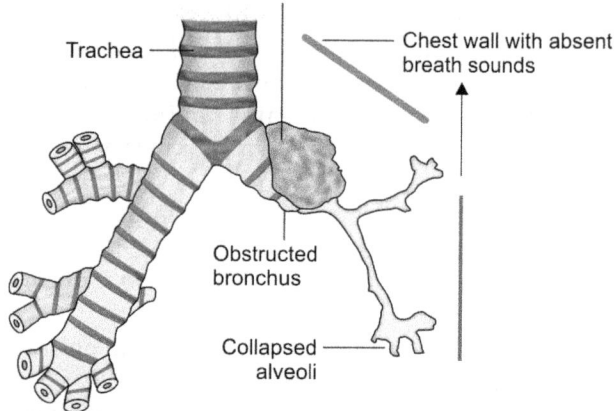

Fig. 2.4: Mass lesion producing collapse of the lung with absent breath sounds on the chest wall

The large mass lesion conducts bronchial breath sounds from the patent bronchus to that part of the chest wall which is in contact with it (usually the supra- and infraclavicular areas)

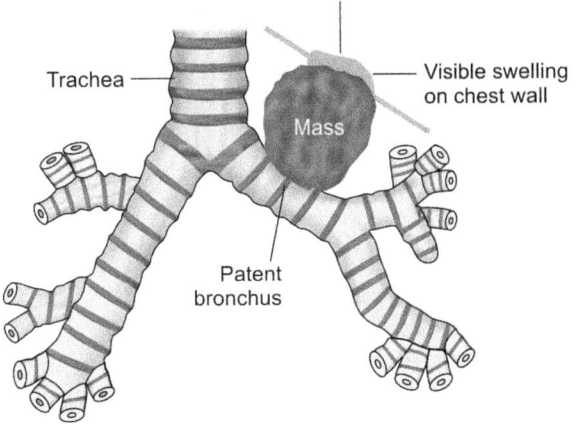

Fig. 2.5: Mass lesion producing bronchial breath sounds on the chest wall

18. Which are the important paraneoplastic syndromes associated with lung malignancy?

The important paraneoplastic syndromes associated with primary lung tumors are the following:

a. Small cell lung cancer is associated with SIADH (leading to hyponatremia), increased ACTH (leading to hypokalemia and muscle weakness), increased melanocyte stimulating hormone (leading to hyperpigmentation) and Lambert-Eaton syndrome.

b. Squamous cell lung cancer is associated with hypercalcemia (leading to lethargy and confusion) and hypoglycemia (due to insulin-like polypeptide).

Some of the other paraneoplastic manifestations are gynecomastia, polyneuropathy, myelopathy, cerebellar degeneration, nephrotic syndrome, polymyositis and dermatomyositis.

19. Which are the malignancies that commonly metastasize to the lungs?

Pulmonary metastases are common and most frequently occur with tumors that have rich systemic venous drainage. The malignancies that commonly metastasize to the lungs are the following:
- Choriocarcinoma
- Renal cell carcinoma
- Breast cancer
- Colon cancer
- Testicular teratomas
- Thyroid cancer
- Melanoma

Standard chest radiography (CXR) is usually the initial modality of investigation for detecting pulmonary metastases. Pulmonary metastases are usually multiple. Radiologically, they vary in size from 3 mm to 15 cm or more (e.g. large cannon-ball lesions). Metastatic pulmonary nodules of the same size are believed to originate at the same time, in a single shower of emboli, and are found most commonly in the outer third of the lungs, especially in the subpleural regions of the lower zones.

20. What is the surface anatomy of various lung lobes?

The surface anatomy of the various lung lobes are important in localizing the disease process to a particular lobe based on the clinical signs elicited on examination of the chest wall (Table 2.1 and Fig. 2.6).

Table 2.1: Types of lung lobes

Lobes	Right side	Left side
Upper lobe	• Suprascapular area • Supraclavicular area • Infraclavicular area (up to 3rd rib) • Axillary area (up to 6th rib)	• Suprascapular area • Supraclavicular area • Infraclavicular area (up to the 3rd rib) • Axillary area (up to 6th rib)
Middle lobe	Mammary area (3rd to 6th rib)	
Lower lobe	• Lower lateral mammary area • Lower axillary area (posteriorly) • Infra-axillary (6th to 8th rib) area • Interscapular area • Subscapular area (up to 12th rib)	• Lower lateral mammary area • Lower axillary area (posteriorly) • Infra-axillary (6th to 8th rib) area • Interscapular area • Subscapular area (up to 12th rib)

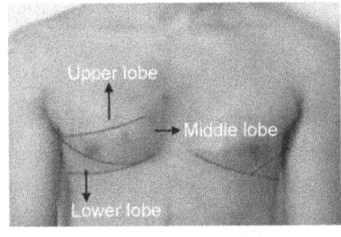
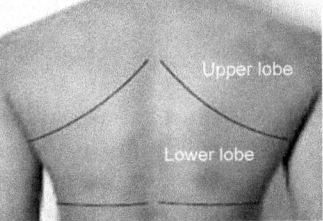

Fig. 2.6: Surface anatomy of anterior and posterior chest wall

The ideal position for examining the respiratory system is the sitting position. The corresponding areas on either side of the chest wall should be examined and compared.

21. **What is meant by vocal fremitus or tactile fremitus?**
    Vibrations which are generated in the larynx (when the patient speaks) are transmitted through the bronchopulmonary system to the chest wall and these vibrations are palpated with the ulnar surface of the examiner's hand. These palpable vibrations are referred to as the tactile vocal fremitus (Fig. 2.7).

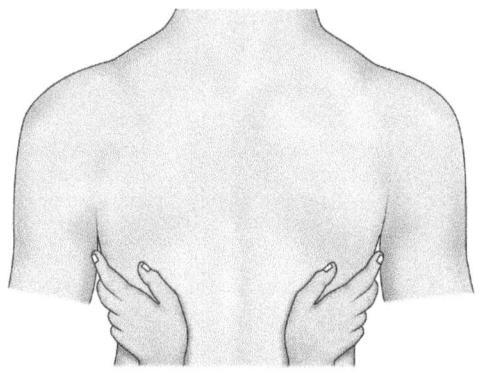

Fig. 2.7: Eliciting vocal fremitus

22. **What are the factors influencing vocal fremitus?**
    Vocal fremitus is decreased or absent when the voice is soft or when the transmission of vibrations from the larynx to the surface of the chest is impeded by an obstructed bronchus, or by the separation of the pleural surfaces by fluid (pleural effusion) or air (pneumothorax). Pleural thickening in conditions like fibrothorax and very thick chest wall also causes decreased vocal fremitus.

    Vocal fremitus is increased when the conduction of vibrations to the chest wall is increased through solidified lung tissue as in consolidation.

Chapter 3
Chest Percussion

1. What are the various factors that influence the chest percussion note?

Resonance is the percussion note obtained during percussion of the normal lung and it is influenced by various factors. It is important to remember that lesions that are more than 5 cm away from the chest wall or those that are less than 3 cm in diameter will not produce any alteration to the normal percussion note.

Dullness replaces resonance when fluid or solid tissue replaces the air within the alveoli or occupies the pleural space in between the two layers of pleura. This occurs in conditions like lobar pneumonia (because the alveoli are filled with secretions) and also in pleural effusion, hemothorax and empyema. In pleural fibrosis there is thickening of the pleural membranes thereby resulting in a dull or impaired percussion note (Fig. 3.1).

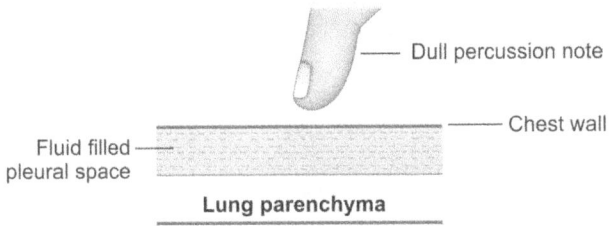

Fig. 3.1: Dull percussion note in pleural effusion

In conditions like emphysema or asthma, generalized hyperresonance during percussion may be heard over the hyperinflated lungs. Unilateral hyperresonance suggests a large pneumothorax or a large air filled bulla in the lung which is close to the chest wall (Fig. 3.2).

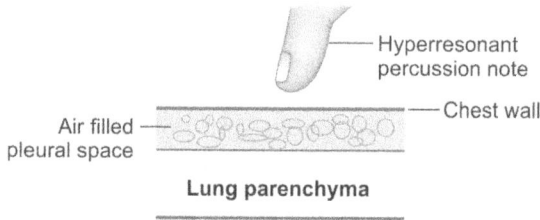

Fig. 3.2: Hyperresonant percussion note in pneumothorax

2. What are the different types of percussion note?

The first step in percussion of the lungs is the comparative percussion of both the anterior and posterior lung fields. Comparative percussion is based on the comparison of sounds elicited at both sides of a symmetrical organ. Normal aerated lung tissue will produce the resonant percussion note (Fig. 3.3 and Box 3.1).

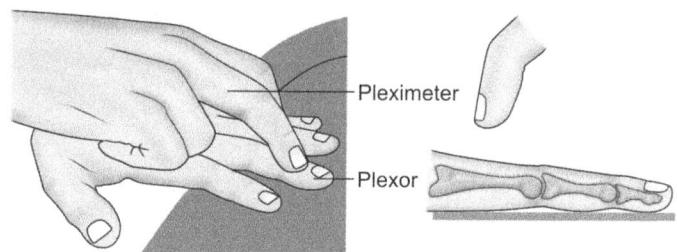

Fig. 3.3: Chest percussion (the blow on the plexor should come from the wrist joint)

> **Box 3.1:** Types of chest percussion notes
>
> - Tympanitic note is a drum-like note elicited over gas containing hollow viscera-like stomach
> - Hyperresonant note is the note elicited over a pneumothorax, large cavity, bullae or emphysema
> - Impaired or dull note is the note elicited over a relatively airless lung as in consolidation, fibrosis or collapse
> - Stony dull note is an extreme form of dull note as one would experience when percussing over a stone, and it is seen in conditions like pleural effusion or a large solid lung tumor.

3. What is significance of the Kronig's isthmus?

This is a band-shaped area of normal lung resonance usually about 5 cm in width in the supraclavicular region located in between the structures at the root of the neck and the shoulder joint. This band of resonance connects the large zones of lung resonance over the anterior and posterior aspects of each side of chest. Dullness in the area of Kronig's isthmus is suggestive of apical segment pathology like tuberculosis or superior sulcus tumor (Pancoast tumor) (Fig. 3.4).

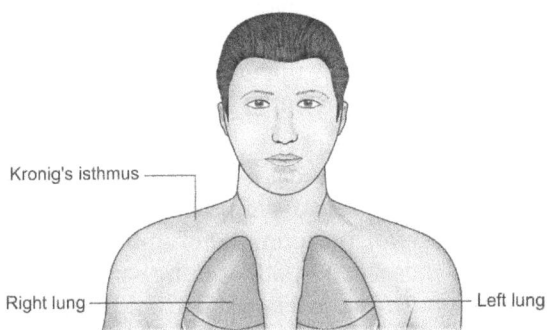

Fig. 3.4: Kronig's isthmus

4. What is Pancoast syndrome?

Pancoast syndrome is caused either by a superior sulcus tumor (squamous cell tumor) or a superior sulcus infiltrative disorder like apical tuberculosis. The syndrome presents with the following features (Box 3.2).

> **Box 3.2:** Clinical features of Pancoast syndrome
>
> - Radicular pain along the ulnar side of upper limb—due to C8, T1 infiltration
> - Small muscle wasting of the hand–due to C8, T1 infiltration
> - Horner's syndrome—due to thoracic symphathetic chain infiltration
> - Chest pain—due to rib erosion

5. What are the features of cervical rib or thoracic outlet syndrome?

Angulation of the fibers from C8 and T1 roots entering the brachial plexus over an abnormal cervical rib or a fibrous band extending from C7 to the first rib, can cause wasting and weakness in the hand and medial forearm along with paresthesias (called as the neurogenic thoracic outlet syndrome). Similarly, angulation of the subclavian artery over an abnormal rib may cause Raynaud's phenomenon, aneurysmal dilatation and embolic events in the upper limb on that side (called as the vascular thoracic outlet syndrome).

6. What is Adson's test?

Adson's test is a clinical test to demonstrate thoracic outlet obstruction in a symptomatic patient. With the patient in sitting position, the examiner palpates both the radial pulses of the patient as the patient takes a deep inspiration. The patient is asked to hold his breath at the end of inspiration. Now with the breath held, the patient hyperextends his neck and turns his head towards the 'affected' side. While doing this, if the examiner feels that the radial pulse of the patient on that side is diminished or obliterated, then the result is considered as positive for thoracic outlet obstruction on that side.

7. Why does mycobacteria predominantly infect the upper lobes of the lung?

The ratio of pulmonary ventilation to pulmonary blood flow for the whole lung at rest is about 0.8. However, there are relatively marked differences in the ventilation to perfusion ratio (V/P ratio) in various parts of the lung as a result of the effect of gravity. Ventilation as well as perfusion declines steadily from the bases to the apices of the lungs. But the decrease in perfusion is much more than the decrease in ventilation and so the V/P ratios are high in the upper portions of the lung. This regional differences in ventilation to perfusion ratio tends to localize some diseases to the upper or lower regions of the lung.

Because of the high V/P ratios in the upper lung areas, there is relatively high alveolar oxygen content (alveolar PO_2) in these areas of the lung. This higher alveolar oxygen content provides a favorable environment for the growth of bacteria like mycobacterium tuberculosis. Tuberculosis typically involves the apical and posterior segments of the upper lobe (85%). A lesion that is confined only to the anterior segment suggests a diagnosis other than tuberculosis (e.g. malignancy).

8. What is meant by Traube's area?

This is a semilunar area of tympanitic resonance at the lower border of the left lung anteriorly. This area of tympanitic resonance is bounded above by the lower margin of normal lung resonance, on the right by the liver dullness, on the left by the splenic dullness and below by the left costal margin (Fig. 3.5).

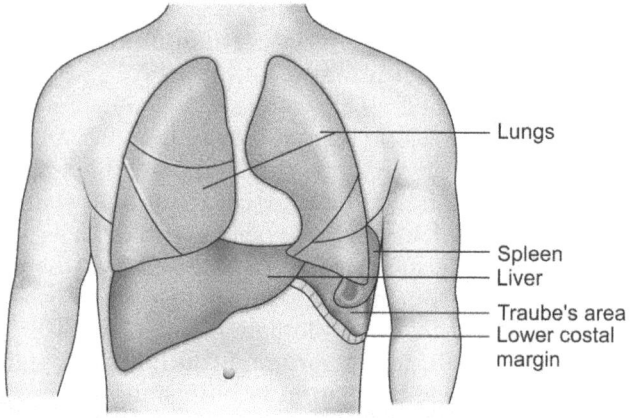

Fig. 3.5: Traube's area

This area is normally occupied by the stomach which gives rise to the tympanitic note. But in large left sided pleural effusion, the diaphragm and the stomach are pushed downwards and this area is occupied by the effusion. So this area becomes dull to percussion. Common conditions producing dullness of this area are the following (Box 3.3):

Box 3.3: Traube's area dullness

- Left-sided pleural effusion
- Left lower lobe consolidation
- Splenomegaly
- Enlarged left lobe of liver
- Ascites
- Tumors of the gastric fundus

9. What is meant by Grocco's and Garland's triangle?

Massive unilateral pleural effusion can cause shift of mediastinum to the opposite side and relaxation of some parts of the lung parenchyma above the effusion. These anatomical factors result in alteration to the normal percussion notes on the posterior chest wall.

Grocco's triangle is a triangular area of dullness located posteriorly on the opposite side of a massive pleural effusion due to shift of posterior mediastinum to that side (Fig. 3.6).

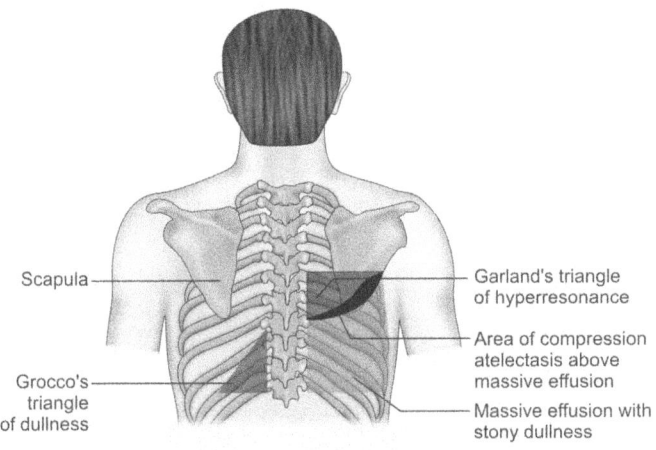

Fig. 3.6: Grocco's and Garland's triangle

Garland's triangle is a triangular area of hyperresonance located posteriorly close to the spine above a large pleural effusion due to "relaxed" lung above the medial part of the effusion (parts of the lung above the lateral part of the effusion are compressed by the effusion causing compression atelectasis). Sometimes, it is possible to elicit a hyperresonant note with a boxy quality in the Garland's triangle, and this phenomenon is referred to as the skodaic resonance.

10. **What is Ewart's sign?**

    Ewart's sign is a physical sign seen in patients with pericardial effusion. Sometimes, a large pericardial effusion may produce an area of dullness near the lower angle of the left scapula. This sign is known as the Ewart's sign (Fig. 3.7).

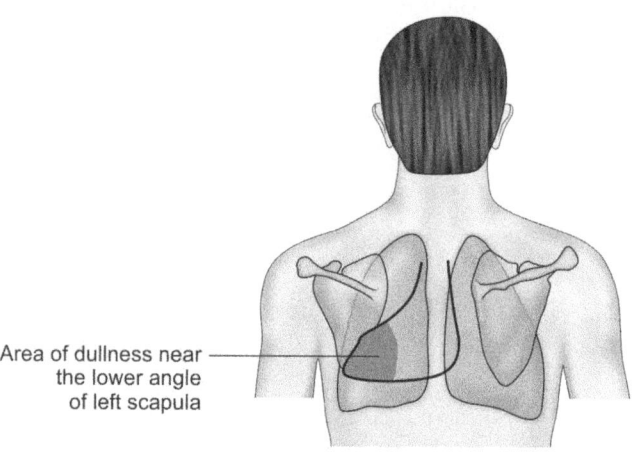

Fig. 3.7: Ewart's sign

11. **What is cracked-pot resonance?**

    This is a type of tympanic resonance which can be elicited normally over the chest of an infant or child during the act of crying. Pathologically, it is found over a lung cavity that is in communication with a bronchus. It is due to the sudden expulsion of air from the cavity into the bronchus, through the narrow opening or communication. The cracked-pot note can be artificially imitated by clasping the hands loosely together and then striking the clasped hand against the knee.

12. What are the non-respiratory causes of unilateral pleural effusion?

Unilateral right-sided pleural effusion is common in hepatic hydrothorax (seen in cirrhosis), Meig's syndrome (pleural effusion associated with ovarian fibroma) and right sided sub-diaphragmatic absess.

Unilateral left sided pleural effusion is common in acute pancreatitis, rupture of oesophagus and left sided subdiaphragmatic abscess. The first two conditions are associated with high level of amylase in the pleural fluid. In acute pancretitis, the effusion results from contact of the pleura with enzyme rich peripancreatic fluid that gains access to the pleural space, most commonly via the transdiaphragmatic lymphatics (Table 3.1).

Table 3.1: Difference between right-sided and left-sided effusion

Right-sided effusion	Left-sided effusion
Hepatic hydrothorax	Acute pancreatitis
Meigs' syndrome	Rupture of esophagus
Right subdiaphragmatic abscess	Left subdiaphragmatic abscess

13. What is the pathogenesis of pleural effusion in generalized systemic disorders?

Normally, fluid enters the pleural space from the capillaries of the parietal pleura and is removed by the lymphatics situated in the parietal pleura. Pleural effusion occurs when the rate of pleural fluid formation exceeds the rate of removal. Pleural effusions due to generalized systemic disorders are often bilateral and are caused by increased rate of fluid formation by any of the following mechanisms:

- **Increased venous pressure** in fluid overload conditions like congestive cardiac failure and hypothyroidism causes bilateral trasudative effusion.
- **Decreased oncotic pressure** in hypoproteinemic conditions like cirrhosis and nephrotic syndrome causes bilateral transudative effusion.
- **Increased capillary permeability** due to inflammation (e.g. in rheumatoid arthritis, SLE, etc.) or delayed hypersensitivity reaction (e.g. drugs like nitrofurantoin, dantrolene, methysergide, bromocriptine, procarbazine, amiodarone, etc.) causes bilateral exudative effusion.

14. What is importance of Light's criteria in pleural effusion?

Light's criteria helps to differentiate an exudative pleural effusion from a transudative effusion. If atleast one of the Light's criteria (Box 3.4) is present, then the effusion is considered as exudative. Transudative pleural effusions meet none of the Light's criteria.

Box 3.4: Light's criteria

- Pleural fluid protein/serum protein = >0.5
- Pleural fluid LDH/serum LDH = >0.6
- Pleural fluid LDH more than two thirds of the normal upper limit of serum LDH

LDH (lactate dehydrogenase) is an enzyme that is released from inflamed and injured pleural tissue. A pseudoexudate is actually a transudative effusion which meets one or more of the Light's criteria. It is seen in diuretic treated cases of heart failure, cirrhosis or nephrotic syndrome.

15. What are the most common types of exudative and transudative pleural effusions?

The most common type of exudative pleural effusion is parapneumonic effusion. About 40% of patients hospitalized with pneumonia have parapneumonic or synpneumonic pleural effusion. The most common cause of transudative pleural effusion is congestive cardiac failure. Pleural effusion in congestive heart failure is usually bilateral. If unilateral, then it is found more often on the right side. This is supposed to be due to the larger pleural surface of the right lung predisposing to transudation of more fluid into the pleural cavity.

16. What is a phantom tumor?

In congestive cardiac failure an interlobar effusion may sometimes develop and this is referred to as the "phantom tumor". This interlobar effusion disappears after diuretic therapy. Hence, it is also called as the "vanishing tumor".

17. What are the features of a complicated synpneumonic or parapneumonic pleural effusion?

Pleural effusion is seen in about 40% of pneumonias. Most of them resolve spontaneously with the successful treatment of pneumonia. However, if the pleural fluid analysis shows any of the following features (Box 3.5), then it is a complicated synpneumonic effusion and is an indication for tube thoracostomy.

> **Box 3.5:** Features of complicated synpneumonic effusion
>
> - Presence of bacteria on gram-stained films of the pleural fluid
> - Pleural fluid pH less than 7.2
> - Pleural fluid glucose less than 60 mg/dL
> - Presence of pus in the pleural cavity

The pleural fluid glucose concentration and pH usually go together (i.e. if glucose is low, then pH also is low). Glucose levels are low in rheumatoid effusion, malignant mesothelioma and empyema.

18. What is meant by re-expansion pulmonary edema?

Re-expansion pulmonary edema represents a form of unilateral pulmonary edema that occurs following the rapid evacuation of fluid or air from the ipsilateral pleural space. In most cases, the hydrothorax or pneumothorax is large in volume and has been present for several days (so it is unusual to occur in emergency situations like tension pneumothorax).

Re-expansion pulmonary edema is due to the sudden increase in the negative intrapleural pressure which leads to alterations in the alveolar surface tension and increased capillary permeability. This in turn results in sudden pulmonary edema.

Re-expansion pulmonary edema can be prevented by the slow withdrawl of pleural fluid or air. Therapeutic aspiration may be required to palliate breathlessness, but removing more than 1.5 liters of pleural fluid in one session is inadvisable as there is risk of re-expansion pulmonary edema.

19. What are the characteristics of a tuberculous pleural effusion?

Tuberculosis continues to be one of the most common cause of pleural effusion even in the absence of demonstrable pulmonary parenchymal lesions on the chest X-ray. The current hypothesis for the pathogenesis of primary tuberculous pleural effusion is that a subpleural caseous focus in the lung ruptures into the pleural space 6 to 12 weeks after the primary infection.

This allows tuberculous protein to enter the pleural space and this in turn generates a delayed hypersensitivity reaction. This reaction is responsible for most of the clinical manifestations including accumulation of fluid in the pleural space. This hypothesis is supported by the fact that cultures of pleural specimens from patients with tuberculous pleurisy are frequently negative for mycobacteria. Some of the features that help in the diagnosis of a tuberculous pleural effusion are the following (Box 3.6):

> **Box 3.6:** Features of tuberculous pleural effusion
> - Presence of caseous granulomas in biopsies of the parietal pleura (at least 4 biopsies should be taken from 4 different sites)
> - Exudative lymphocyte predominant effusion with low glucose content
> - High levels of adenosine deaminase enzyme in the pleural fluid. The ADA 1 isomer is nonspecific and may be elevated in empyema, rheumatoid effusion, etc. But the ADA 2 isomer is relatively specific for tuberculous effusion
> - High level of interferon gamma in pleural fluid
> - Pleural thickening (of more than 1 cm) on computed tomography (CT)

Tuberculous pleurisy responds well to medical therapy. Therapeutic drainage of tuberculous effusion is recommended only if the effusion is causing discomfort. There is usually rapid response to antituberculous drugs with no need for aspiration. Resorption of the pleural fluid occurs within 6 to 12 weeks of starting antituberculous treatment. The addition of corticosteroids may lead to more rapid resolution of symptoms and pleural fluid on the chest radiograph. Some of the rare complications include bronchopleural fistula, empyema and fibrothorax.

20. What is the role of empirical ATT in a suspected case of tuberculous pleural effusion?

Empiric antituberculous therapy is appropriate in certain patients. A positive tuberculin skin test in a patient less than 40-year-old, in combination with a pleural fluid analysis that is compatible with tuberculosis, is an indication for empiric antituberculous therapy. In contrast, a patient with a suspected tuberculous pleural effusion who is more than 40-year-old and who has risk factors for bronchogenic carcinoma should be subjected to thoracoscopy or open pleural biopsy rather than to empiric therapy (*Ref: Fishman's Pulmonary Diseases and Disorders; 4th edition*).

The absence of granulomatous inflammation in the open pleural biopsy of a tuberculin skin test positive patient virtually excludes the diagnosis of tuberculosis and obviates the need for antituberculous therapy.

21. What is paramalignant or paraneoplastic pleural effusion?

Patients with malignancy can develop pleural effusion even when tumor cells are absent from the pleural space. This occurs due to indirect effects of the neoplasm like hypoalbuminemia which produces transudative pleural effusion. This type of effusion is called paramalignant or paraneoplastic pleural effusion.

22. What are the clinical features of empyema?

Empyema means pus in the pleural cavity. Clinical features suggesting possibility of empyema are the following (Box 3.7):

> **Box 3.7:** Clinical features of empyema
>
> - Severe pleuritic chest pain
> - High grade fever with chills
> - Clubbing of fingers (may develop in 10–14 days)
> - Fullness of intercostal spaces with overlying tense erythematous skin and tenderness during palpation and percussion of the chest wall

Presence of empyema is an indication for tube thoracostomy. If the pus is thick or if the pus is multiloculated, then thoracotomy with decortication is needed.

23. Which is the ideal site for chest tube insertion?

Chest drain insertion should be done in the "triangle of safety". This is the triangle bordered by the anterior border of the latissimus dorsi, the lateral border of the pectoralis major muscle and a line parallel to the horizontal level of the nipple. The triangle has its apex in the axilla (Fig. 3.8).

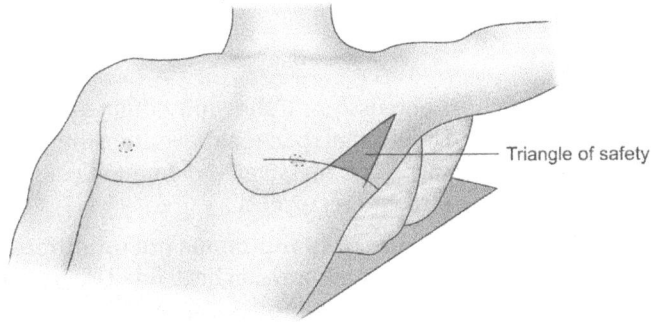

Fig. 3.8: Triangle of safety

The preferred position of the patient for chest drain insertion is lying on the bed (as shown in Fig. 3.8), with the arm on the side of the lesion behind the patient's head. This position ensures that the axillary area is well exposed. Chest tubes are typically left in place until the drainage rate has fallen below 50 mL per day.

24. How much fliud is needed for clinical detection of pleural effusion?

In healthy adults, the pleural space contains normally about 10 mL of pleural fluid at any one time. To diagnose pleural effusion clinically, there should be a minimum of 500 mL of fluid in the pleural cavity. The minimum amount of fluid required for the clinical detection of fluid in the various body cavities are as follows (Table 3.2).

Table 3.2: Minimum amount of fluid is needed for clinical detection of pleural effusion

Body cavity	Method of elicitation	Minimum fluid
Pleural cavity	Chest percussion	500 mL
Abdominal cavity	Shifting dullness	1,000 mL
	Fluid thrill	2,000 mL
	Puddle sign	120 mL

On chest percussion, if the stony dullness extends upto the 2nd intercostal space or above, then the effusion is clinically said to be massive. Malignant effusions are usually massive and recurrent.

25. What are the types of spontaneous pneumothorax?

Spontaneous pneumothorax can be divided into primary and secondary pneumothorax. Primary spontaneous pneumothorax occurs in otherwise healthy persons. Secondary spontaneous pneumothorax occurs in persons with underlying lung disease. The most common cause of secondary spontaneous pneumothorax is emphysema.

26. How is pneumothorax classified based on the mechanism of air trapping?

Based on the mechanism of air trapping there are three types of pneumothorax. They are the following:

- Closed pneumothorax: It is usually due to the rupture of sub-pleural blebs. In this type, the communication between the pleural cavity and the lung seals off spontaneously and the trapped air within the pleural cavity is slowly reabsorbed (1.25% of hemithorax volume per day). So a small closed spontaneous pneumothorax (less than 15% of hemithorax) may be observed without active intervention, if the patient is asymptomatic.
- Open pneumothorax: It usually follows rupture of a bullae or lung abscess. In this type the communication between the pleural cavity and the lung remains patent and air can move to and fro through this bronchopleural fistula. This type of pneumothorax can lead to hydro or pyopneumothorax. Surgical closure of the fistula should be done.
- Tension pneumothorax: In this type, the communication between the pleural cavity and the lung remains patent and acts like a one way valve, allowing the passage of air only into the pleural cavity. This causes large amount of air trapping within the pleural cavity and leads to the collapse of the underlying lung. This is a medical emergency and should be treated by inserting a water seal intercostal drainage system into the pleural cavity.

27. What is catamenial pneumothorax?

Catamenial pneumothorax (thoracic endometriosis syndrome) occurs in relation to the menstrual cycle and usually is recurrent. It typically occurs in women who are 30–40 years of age and have a history of endometriosis.

It usually affects the right lung and develops within 72 hours of onset of menstruation. Although, the cause of catamenial pneumothorax is unknown, it has been suggested that air may gain access to the peritoneal cavity during menstruation. This air then enters the pleural cavity through a diaphragmatic defect causing pneumothorax.

28. What is meant by shifting dullness?

In conditions like hydropneumothorax or a large fluid filled superficial lung cavity, the upper border of dullness is horizontal and is sharply confined to a particular intercostal space (anteriorly, laterally and posteriorly) and this can be marked out by percussing the chest wall in the sitting position. Changing the patient to the supine position leads to gravity dependant fluid shifting and this can cause the previously dull intercostal space to become resonant. This phenomenon is called as shifting dullness (Figs 3.9A and B).

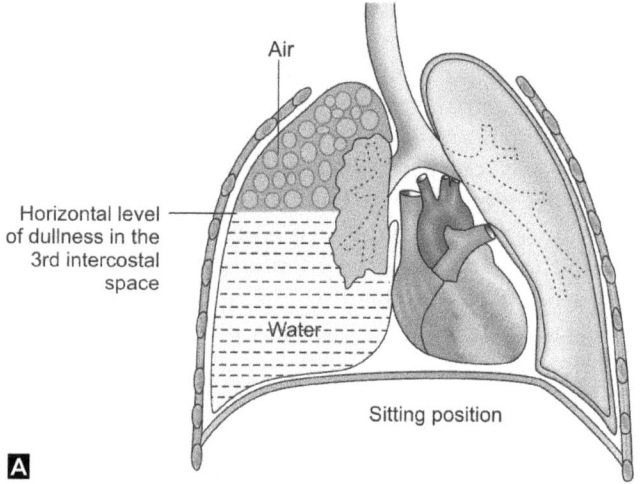

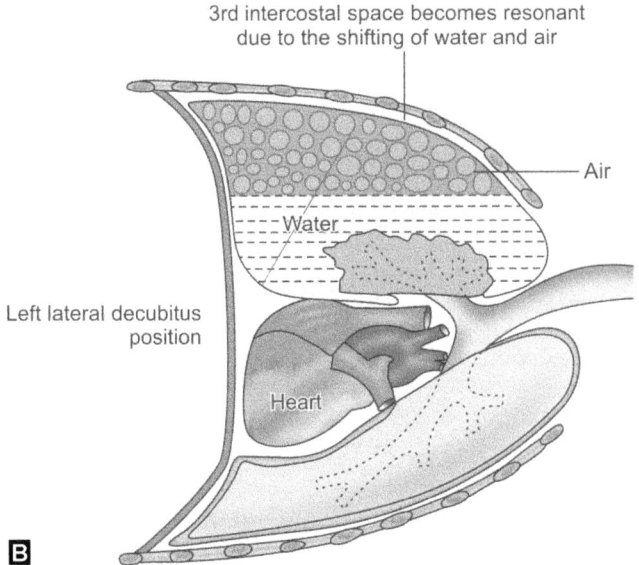

Figs 3.9A and B: Demonstration of shifting dullness

29. What is tidal percussion?

Normally, during deep inspiration, as the lungs expand, the diaphragm moves down and the area of lung resonance also move downwards by about 4 cm (approximately one intercostal space). This downward increase in the area of resonance can be demonstrated by percussing out the lower margin of lung resonance at the beginning and at the end of a deep inspiration (either anteriorly along the mid-clavicular line or posteriorly along the scapular line) and by noting the difference between the two levels. This is called as tidal percussion (Fig. 3.10).

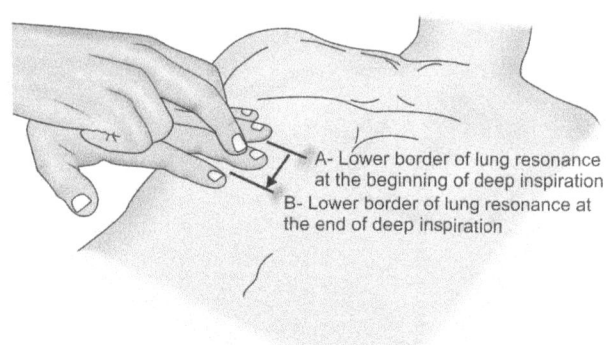

Fig. 3.10: Tidal percussion

30. What is the clinical relevance of tidal percussion?

A dull or impaired percussion note obtained in the lower intercostal spaces may be due to subdiaphragmatic pathology or lower lobe pathology. Tidal percussion helps to differentiate between these two entities.

In subdiaphragmatic pathology, the lung usually expands normally and so the downward increase in the area of lung resonance during deep inspiration is almost normal (about 4 cm or one intercostal space). But in lower lobe pathologies like consolidation or effusion, the normal lung expansion is compromised. Hence no downward increase in the area of lung resonance can be demonstrated by tidal percussion in such situations. Tidal percussion also helps to assess the mobility of the diaphragm.

Chapter
4   Auscultation of the Chest

1. How are the normal breath sounds produced?

Breath sounds are produced by the vibration of vocal cords due to the turbulent flow of air through the larynx and they are high pitched at the sites of their origin. High pitched sounds are perceived as loud sounds. These high pitched sounds are then transmitted along the trachea and bronchi to the chest wall and during this process they are filtered and muffled by the surrounding air-filled lung tissue (Fig. 4.1).

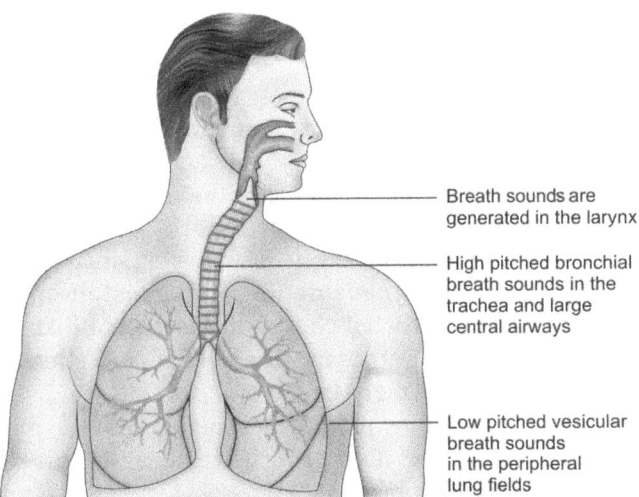

Fig. 4.1: Breath sounds in various locations

Thus, the high pitched sounds generated in the larynx are converted to low pitched sounds and these low pitched sounds are heard over most regions of the chest wall during auscultation. The normal breath sounds are broadly classified into bronchial and vesicular sounds.

2. What are vesicular breath sounds?

Vesicular sounds are soft, breezy, low pitched sounds with a **rustling** quality that are normally heard all over the peripheral lung fields. They are prominent during inspiration and early part of expiration, and there is no silent gap in between the two phases of respiration (Fig. 4.2).

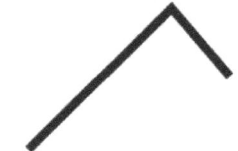

Fig. 4.2: Vesicular breath sound

3. What are the variations that can occur to vesicular breath sounds?

Some disease states can alter the quality of vesicular breath sounds. Vesicular breath sounds may be diminished in intensity in the following situations.

- Conditions causing under-expansion of lungs due to restricted chest wall movement (like chest pain, respiratory muscle weakness, ascites, large abdominal mass, etc.)
- In conditions producing separation of the pleural surfaces by fluid or air (like pleural effusion or pneumothorax)

- In case of pleural thickening due to fibrosis or metastatic infiltrating tumors
- In persons with very thick chest wall.

Vesicular breath sounds with prolonged expiration may be heard in obstructive airway disorders like bronchial asthma and COPD.

4. What are bronchial breath sounds?

Bronchial sounds are loud, harsh, usually high pitched sounds heard normally over the trachea, upper sternum and paraspinal areas upto the second thoracic vertebrae. They are more prominent during expiration and the duration of expiration is equal to or more than that of inspiration. There is a silent gap in between the two phases of respiration (Fig. 4.3 and Table 4.1).

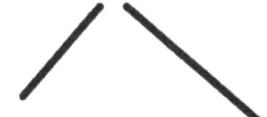

Fig. 4.3: Bronchial breath sound

Table 4.1: Difference between vesicular and bronchial breath sound

Vesicular breath sound	Bronchial breath sound
Soft, breezy and low-pitched	Loud, harsh and high-pitched
Prominent during inspiration	Prominent during expiration
No gap between the two phases	Silent gap between the two phases
Heard over peripheral lung fields	Heard over larger airways

5. What are the types of bronchial breath sounds?

Bronchial breath sounds are considered abnormal when they are heard at locations where vesicular breath sounds are usually heard. There are three types of bronchial breath sounds. They are the following (Box 4.1):

Box 4.1: Types of bronchial breath sounds

- Tubular
- Cavernous
- Amphoric
---

6. What is tubular bronchial breath sound?

Tubular bronchial breath sound is the most common type of bronchial breath sound. It is heard in situations where there is conduction of breath sounds directly from the peripheral bronchi to the overlying chest wall through an interposed solidified lung tissue without the normal filteration or modification by air-filled alveoli.

Such situations occur when consolidated or fibrosed lung tissue or a mass lesion or an area of compression atelectasis (above the level of a massive pleural effusion) is interposed in between a large bronchus and the chest wall. Then the tubular bronchial breath sounds generated in the bronchus are conducted directly to the chest wall without filteration.

7. What is D'Espine's sign?

Sometimes large posterior mediastinal masses may transmit the bronchial breath sounds generated in the large central airways directly to the posterior chest wall. Hence, tubular bronchial breath sounds may be heard in the interscapular area below the second thoracic vertebrae. This sign is called as the D' Espine's sign (Box 4.2).

> **Box 4.2:** Common tumors of the posterior mediastinum
>
> - Neurogenic tumors (Neurofibroma, ganglioneuroma, etc.)
> - Lymphatic tumors
> - Vascular lesions

8. What is cavernous bronchial breath sound?

Cavernous breath sound is a relatively low pitched bronchial breath sound that is heard over a superficial collapsible cavity (more than 2 cm in diameter) with a communicating patent bronchus. Usually such cavities are surrounded by either consolidated or fibrosed lung tissue.

The high pitched tubular bronchial breath sound generated in the bronchus harmonicates within the cavity and is converted to low pitched cavernous bronchial breath sound. This low pitched sound is then conducted to the chestwall by the relatively airless consolidated or fibrosed lung tissue surrounding the cavity (Box 4.3).

> **Box 4.3:** Auscultatory triad of a cavity
>
> - Cavernous bronchial breath sounds
> - Post-tussive suction sound
> - Increased vocal resonance (whispering pectoriloquy)

9. What is amphoric bronchial breath sound?

Amphoric bronchial breath sound is another type of low pitched bronchial breath sound which has high-pitched overtones. It is heard in the case of a very large cavity communicating with a patent bronchus or in cases with bronchopleural fistula. The mechanism of production is the same as that of cavernous bronchial breath sound. However, in this case, some of the reflected sound waves from the walls of the large cavity are high pitched.

10. What is a bronchopleural fistula?

A bronchopleural fistula is a communication between the pleural space and the bronchial tree. It is a rare, but serious complication associated with several pulmonary conditions. In the setting of a spontaneous or non-spontaneous pneumothorax, it is consistent with prolonged air leak. Current American College of Chest Physicians (ACCP) guidelines recommend that, if the air leak persists over 4 days in a case of pneumothorax, then the patient should be considered for surgery to close the air leak.

11. Which are the common adventitious sounds heard during examination of the respiratory system?

The adventitious sounds are broadly classified into continuous and discontinuous sounds. The common continuous sounds are stridor and wheeze (low-pitched wheezes are sometimes referred to as rhonchi). The common discontinuous sounds are the crackle and pleural rub (Table 4.2).

Table 4.2: Adventitious sounds

Continuous sounds	Discontinuous sounds
• Stridor • Wheeze	• Crackle • Pleural rub

12. What is meant by stridor?

Stridor is a high-pitched sound that is produced due to the narrowing or obstruction of the large upper airways i.e. the larynx and the trachea. Stridor is almost always inspiratory (*Ref: Fishman's Pulmonary Diseases and Disorders, 4th edition, Pg 846*). It is best heard over the neck.

The presence of stridor indicates upper airway obstruction and the relief of this obstruction is often a matter of great urgency. Common causes of stridor are a foreign body in the upper intrathoracic airway or esophagus, an acquired lesion of the airway (e.g. carcinoma in adults), or a congenital lesion in children.

13. What is Pickwickian syndrome?

An important cause of stridor in obese people is the obesity hypoventilation syndrome (OHS), or the Pickwickian syndrome. OHS is defined as the **triad** of morbid obesity, day time hypoventilation and sleep disordered breathing in the absence of an alternative neuromuscular, mechanical or metabolic explanation for hypoventilation. Stridor occurs due to the inspiratory pharyngeal collapse in these people. Patients with obesity hypoventilation syndrome often can be confused with patients with COPD since both of these patients manifest daytime hypercapnia. However, patients with COPD have an obstructive pattern on their pulmonary function studies, whereas patients with OHS usually have a restrictive pattern on their pulmonary function studies. In addition, patients with COPD are usually not morbidly obese.

14. What are wheezes and how are they produced?

The American Thoracic Society Committee on pulmonary nomenclature define wheezes as continuous sounds with a dominant frequency of usually 400 Hz or more. There are also lower pitched wheezes with a dominant frequency of 200 Hz or less (these lower pitched sounds were previously referred to as rhonchi). Wheezes are usually more prominent on expiration because the airways tend to become narrower during expiration.

Wheezes are produced by the fluttering or oscillation of adjacent airway walls. At the sites of airway obstruction, airflow velocity reaches a critical value called as the flutter velocity. When airflow attains this critical velocity, the adjacent airway walls begin to flutter or oscillate like the strings of a guitar. This generates the musical sound (Fig. 4.4).

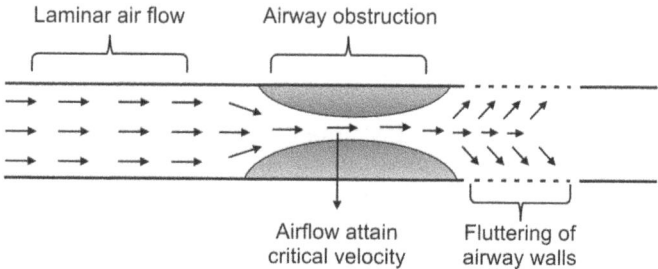

Fig. 4.4: Mechanism of production of wheeze

15. What are the different types of wheeze?

Wheezes are classified as monophonic if the sounds are of the same pitch. Monophonic wheeze suggests localized obstruction of one airway. Wheezes are classified as polyphonic if the sounds are of varying pitch or frequency. Polyphonic wheeze suggests obstruction of airways at multiple sites (Table 4.3).

Table 4.3: Classification of wheeze	
Monophonic wheeze	**Polyphonic wheeze**
Foreign body inhalation	Asthma
Bronchial tumor	COPD

16. What are crackles (rales, crepitations)?

Crackles are discontinuous adventitious breath sounds resembling miniature explosions. They are heard more often during inspiration than during expiration. They may be fine or coarse depending on the mechanism

of production and their timing is of great clinical importance.
- Early inspiratory crackles suggest disease of the small airways
- Late or pan-inspiratory crackles suggest disease of the alveoli.

17. How are fine crackles produced?

In conditions like interstitial fibrosis and in interstitial stage of pulmonary edema, the peripheral airways in the basal territories of the lung remain closed towards the end of expiration. This is due to the following factors:
- Increased elastic recoil of the airways because of the loss of elastic fibers in the interstitium due to interstitial fibrosis
- Due to the compression of the airways by the weight of the overlying fluid filled interstitium in conditions like pulmonary edema.

The air within the alveoli supplied by these closed peripheral airways is considerably below atmospheric pressure. Towards late inspiration, when the intrabronchial pressure increases, these closed peripheral airways eventually reopen. This results in a sudden equalization of pressures across the previously closed parts of these airways. This sudden equalization of pressure produces an explosive sound which is called the fine crackle.

Eventhough crackles are usually associated with diseases of the lung, they can also occur in normal healthy people. Fine late inspiratory crackles may occur in healthy people in the dependent lung regions (i.e. over the anterior lung bases) after prolonged periods of recumbency. These "normal" or "physiological" fine crackles usually resolve after taking few deep inspirations (Figs 4.5 and 4.6).

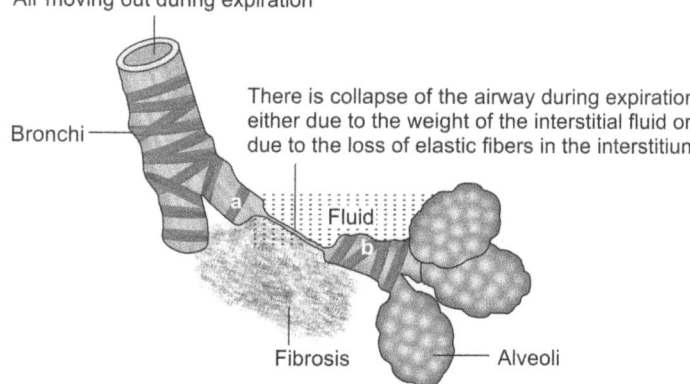

Fig. 4.5: Mechanism of generation of fine crackle—step 1

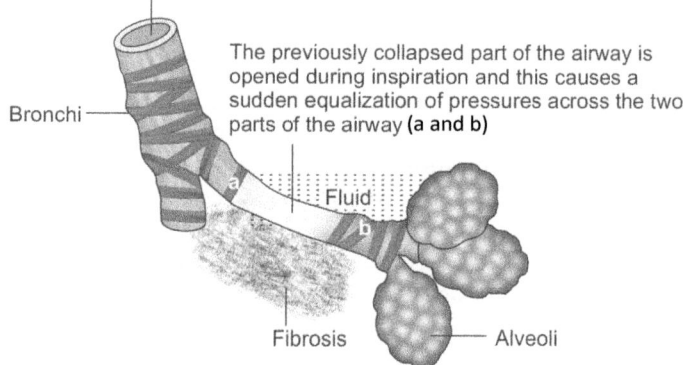

Fig. 4.6 : Mechanism of generation of fine crackle—step 2

18. **What is the effect of gravity on fine crackle?**
    The closure of peripheral airways in the basal territories of the lung in conditions like interstitial edema is mainly due to compression by the weight of the overlying fluid

filled lung. Shifting this fluid by turning a recumbent patient from one side to another can remove this weight and thereby prevent the closure of these peripheral airways. This can result in sudden or gradual disappearance of fine crackles. Hence, fine crackles are said to be gravity dependant and they are not affected by maneuvers like coughing.

19. **What are Velcro crackles?**

    Velcro sounding crackles are a type of fine crackles heard in interstitial fibrosis. They have a distinctive character and are also described as "close to the ear" or "cellophane" crackles. Their sound is similar to the sound of hair rubbed between the fingers. In mild or early stages of interstitial lung disease, they are late inspiratory and are best heard at the basal areas of the lung, with the patient sitting upright. As the disease progresses, these fine crackles may become pan-inspiratory and may extend to higher levels above the lung bases (Box 4.4).

    > **Box 4.4:** Clinical features of interstitial lung disease (ILD)
    > - History of progressive dyspnea
    > - Central cyanosis
    > - Clubbing
    > - Diminished chest movements
    > - Impaired chest percussion note
    > - Velcro crackles

20. **How are coarse crackles produced?**

    Coarse crackles are produced by the passage of boluses of air through an intermittently obstructed airway (usually with thick viscid mucus). The passage of each bolus of air leads to sudden equalization of pressures on either side of the occluded part of the airway. This in turn produces an explosive sound which is the coarse crackle (Fig. 4.7).

They are usually early inspiratory (seen in bronchitis) but can be pan-inspiratory in some conditions like alveolar stage of acute pulmonary edema and bronchiectasis (*Ref: Lung Sounds, Paul Forgacs*).

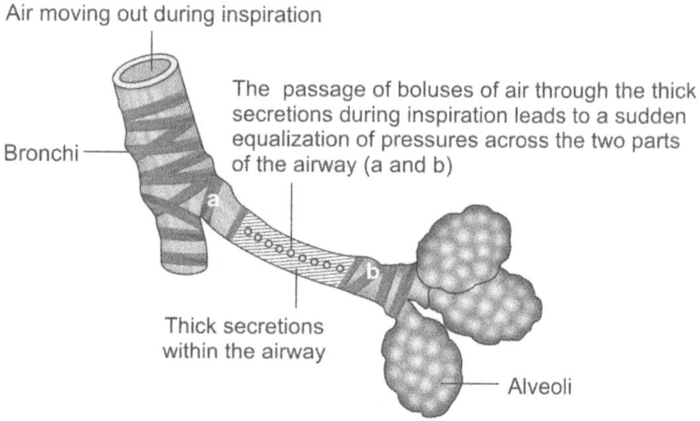

Fig. 4.7: Mechanism of generation of coarse crackle

21. What is the effect of cough on coarse crackle?

The intermittent occlusion of airways which plays an important role in the genesis of the coarse crackle is usually caused by thick mucous secretions within the airway lumen. Coughing causes displacement of these viscid mucous secretions and the airways may remain opened without getting occluded. This in turn may lead to the extinction or disappearance of the coarse crackle, after an act of coughing. So, if coarse crackles are heard, then special attention should be given to appreciate the change in their nature by asking the patient to cough.

22. What are "post-tussive" crackles?

Paradoxically, in early stages of pulmonary tuberculosis, crackles tend to appear in the region of lung apices, after a bout of coughing. This phenomenon is one of the earliest physical signs in this disease. Coughing dislodges the caseous material within the tuberculi infected parenchymal areas of the lung into the adjacent bronchi, producing their transient occlusion. The intermittent passage of air through these occluded bronchi produce the characteristic "post-tussive" crackles.

23. What is pleural rub and how will you differentiate it from crackles?

Pleural rub is a superficial, loud grating sound produced by friction between the two layers of pleura in inflammatory conditions like pleurisy. It is heard during both phases of respiration (predominantly at the end of inspiration or at the beginning of expiration). It is usually a localized sound and the most common site of pleural friction rub is the lower anterolateral chest wall which is the area of greatest thoracic mobility.

Pleural rub can be transiently eliminated by holding the breath (unlike pericardial rub). Pleural rub is not affected by coughing. When the pressure of the stethoscope over the chest wall is increased, the intensity of the rub also increases. The last two features help to differentiate it from crackles (Table 4.4).

Table 4.4: Difference between pleural rub and crackle

Pleural rub	Crackle
Not affected by cough	Affected by cough
Intensity increased by applying more pressure with stethoscope	Applying more pressure with stethoscope has no effect

24. What is the effect of aging on breath sounds?

Variation in breath sounds with aging have long been well documented. This is mainly attributed to the loss of pulmonary elasticity. In otherwise healthy old people, fine crackles can sometimes normally be heard over the lung bases. But these crackles tend to disappear after taking few deep breaths and they have no clinical significance. The recognition of age-related crackles is important because such clinically unimportant crackles are so common among elderly people.

25. What are the auscultatory findings in different types of pulmonary fibrosis?

The breath sounds that are heard in a patient with fibrosis depends on the type of pulmonary fibrosis and the presence or absence of a patent bronchus in the vicinity of fibrosis. However, fine inspiratory crackles are common to all type of fibrosis.

In conditions like tuberculosis, necrotizing pneumonias, pulmonary infarction and radiation exposure, fibrous tissue replaces the damaged lung tissue and this fibrosis is usually very dense and localized. This type of fibrosis is called as the replacement fibrosis. In the areas of replacement fibrosis, there is very little air filled alveoli surrounding the large patent bronchi. The thick fibrosis also pulls the large airways like trachea closer to the chest wall. Hence, tubular bronchial breath sounds generated in these large airways are conducted to the chest wall without much filtration. Hence, tubular bronchial breath sounds along with crackles are heard during auscultation. Also the findings are usually localized to a particular area of chest wall (Fig. 4.8).

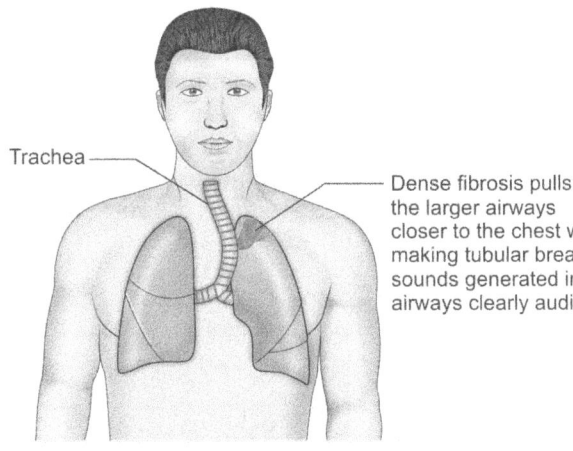

Fig. 4.8: Mechanism of tubular bronchial breath sounds in replacement fibrosis

However, in conditions like idiopathic pulmonary fibrosis, connective tissue diseases and occupational lung diseases, there is widespread interstitial fibrosis which is not dense and focal. So, the bronchi are surrounded by relatively air-filled alveoli (which filters the breath sounds), until the very late stages of the disease. Hence, vesicular type of breath sounds along with fine inspiratory crackles are heard and these findings are not localized (usually bilateral signs).

26. **What is meant by post-tussive suction?**
Cavity is a gas containing space within the lung with a thick wall (thin walled cavities are called as bullae). Post-tussive suction sound is the most definite clinical sign of a superficial, large, collapsible cavity communicating with

a patent bronchus. This is a low-pitched "sucking" sound heard during the long inspiratory phase that follows a bout of coughing. During coughing, the negative pressure generated in the bronchus causes the cavity to collapse, thereby emptying it of its air content. Re-entry of air into this empty cavity from the bronchus during the post-tussive inspiratory phase produces the sucking sound (Figs 4.9A and B).

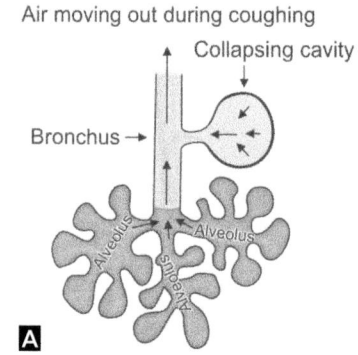

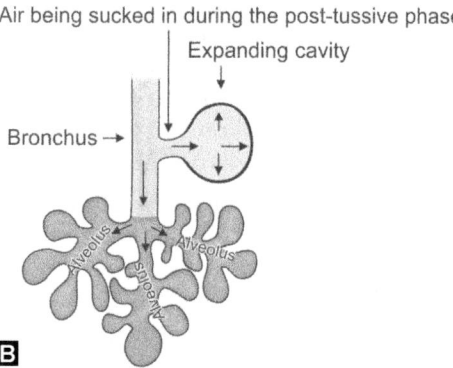

Figs 4.9A and B: Mechanism of generation of post-tussive suction sound

27. What is meant by succussion splash?

Succussion splash is a "splashing" sound heard over the chest wall when the chest of a patient is shaken suddenly. If heard, it is always abnormal. It is seen in the following conditions:
- Hydropneumothorax
- Large fluid filled lung cavity
- Herniation of stomach or colon into the thoracic cavity

The most common cause of hydropneumothorax is iatrogenic (following aspiration of pleural effusion). Other causes of hydropneumothorax are trauma (hemopneumothorax) and rupture of subpleural abscess (pyopneumothorax).

28. What are the important causes of cavitation within the lungs?

A cavity has been defined pathologically as "a gas-filled space within a zone of consolidation, mass or nodule in the lung". The most important causes of cavitation in the lungs are the following (Box 4.5):

Box 4.5: Diseases associated with lung cavity

- Malignancy (usually squamous cell carcinoma)
- Lung abscess (staphylococci and *Klebsiella*)
- Tuberculosis (progressive primary and secondary)
- Fungal infections
- Hydatid cyst
- Congenital cysts
- Traumatic cysts
- Wegener's granulomatosis
- Cystic bronchiectasis
- Pulmonary infarction

29. What do you know about the formation of a tuberculous cavity?

Cavity is the characteristic lesion of post-primary pulmonary tuberculosis. Post-primary tuberculosis may be the result of either endogenous reactivation of latent foci of tuberculous infection or exogenous re-infection. The characteristic feature of post-primary pulmonary tuberculosis is gross tissue necrosis. This results in the formation of large lesions containing abundant caseous necrotic tissue called as tuberculomas. The central part of the tuberculoma is anoxic and acidic, and provides a hostile environment to the tubercle bacilli. The caseous material in the center of the tuberculoma is softened and eventually liquefied by proteases secreted by activated macrophages. The enlarging tuberculoma eventually erodes into a bronchus and discharges the softened caseous material into the bronchial tree. This results in the formation of a tuberculous cavity.

The environment in the cavity is quite different from that of the closed tuberculoma. Air enriched with carbon dioxide enters the cavity and neutralizes the acidity and provides oxygen for the tubercle bacilli. The bacilli are then able to replicate freely. When these bacilli gain access to the bronchi and are expectorated in the sputum, the patient becomes infectious and is said to have "open tuberculosis". Bacilli escaping from the cavities may infect other parts of the same lung or the other lung by endobronchial spread.

30. What is egophony or 'E' to 'A' sign and why is it elicited above the level of a massive pleural effusion?

Egophony is an extreme form of increased vocal resonance where the words spoken by the patient, when heard by the examiner, have a nasal or bleating quality, due to change in timbre of the voice (Fig. 4.10).

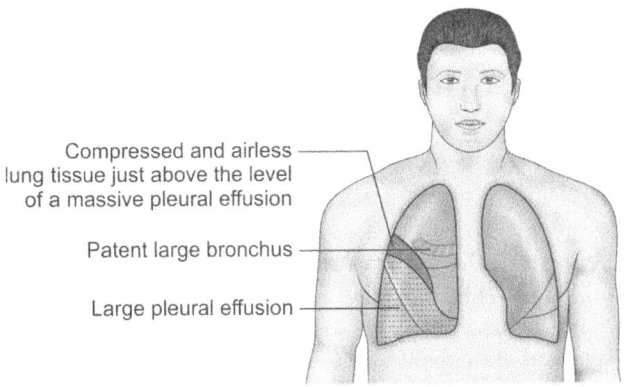

Fig. 4.10: E to A sign in massive pleural effusion

Parts of the lung tissue lying close to the upper margin of a massive pleural effusion are actually compressed by the effusion. This compression make these parts of the lung airless and they behave like a solidified lung tissue (also called as compression atelectasis). So, this compressed part of the lung transmits tubular bronchial breath sounds from a nearby patent bronchus directly to the chest wall. Hence, tubular bronchial breath sounds and increased vocal resonance in the form of egophony are elicited above the level of a massive pleural effusion (on the posterolateral chest wall). Egophony is also seen in areas of consolidation.

31. Which are the clinical signs that always go together during examination of the respiratory system?

The **three** physical signs that always go together are (1) increased vocal fremitus, (2) bronchial breath sounds and (3) increased vocal resonance. This is because all of them are due to identical mechanism, i.e. increased transmission of the sound vibrations or waves through solidified and airless lung tissue to the chest wall (e.g. as in a case of consolidation of lung).

Chapter 5
Interstitial Lung Diseases

1. What are the commonest causes of interstitial lung disease (ILD)?

The interstitial lung diseases are characterized by clinical changes consistent with restrictive rather than obstructive changes in the lung. Persons with interstitial lung diseases have dyspnea, tachypnea, and eventual cyanosis, without evidence of wheezing or signs of airway obstruction. Usually, there is an insidious onset of breathlessness that initially occurs during exercise and may progress to the point at which the person is totally incapacitated. Fine **inspiratory crackles and clubbing are usually present**. The commonest causes of ILD are the following:

- Idiopathic pulmonary fibrosis (IPF)—usually affects elderly people
- Sarcoidosis
- Interstitial lung disease associated with collagen vascular disease
    - Systemic lupus erythematosus (SLE)—shrinking lungs
    - Rheumatoid arthritis
- Pneumoconiosis
    - Asbestosis
    - Silicosis
    - Coal worker's pneumoconiosis, etc.

2. What is the pathogenesis of fibrosis in interstitial lung diseases?

Current theory suggests that most interstitial lung diseases, regardless of the causes, have a common pathogenesis. In contrast to the obstructive lung diseases, which primarily involve the airways of the lung, the interstitial lung disorders exert their effects on the collagen and elastic connective tissue found between the airways and the blood vessels of the lung.

It is thought that these disorders are initiated by some type of injury to the alveolar epithelium, followed by an inflammatory process that involves the alveoli and interstitium of the lung. An accumulation of inflammatory and immune cells causes continued damage to lung tissue and replacement of the normal functioning lung tissue with fibrous scar tissue.

3. What are the peculiarities of breathing in a person with stiff lungs due to interstitial fibrosis or edema?

Typically, a person with a stiff lung due to interstitial fibrosis or edema, breathes with a pattern of rapid, shallow respirations. This tachypneic pattern of breathing, in which the respiratory rate is increased and the tidal volume is decreased, reduces the work of breathing. This is because it takes less work to move air through the airways at an increased rate than it does to stretch a stiff lung to accommodate a larger tidal volume.

4. What is meant by pneumoconiosis?

Pneumoconiosis refers to the accumulation of inorganic dust (asbestos, silica, coal mine dust, etc.) in the lungs and the consequences of the tissues response to the presence of the dust. The most dangerous particles are those in the range of 1–5 μm in size (Table 5.1).

Table 5.1: Pneumoconiosis with upper and lower lobe predominance

Upper lobe predominance	Lower lobe predominance
• Berylliosis • Coal worker's pneumoconiosis • Silicosis	• Asbestosis

5. **What are the most common manifestations of asbestos exposure?**

   Pleural disease is the most common manifestation of asbestos exposure. The non-malignant manifestations of asbestos exposure in the pleural space include circumscribed pleural plaques, diffuse pleural thickening, rounded atelectasis and pleural effusions. Asbestos exposure can also result in asbestosis (a type of ILD), malignant mesothelioma of the pleura and adenocarcinoma of the lung.

6. **What is the relationship between tuberculosis and silicosis?**

   The link between silicosis and tuberculosis has been recognized for nearly a century. The ingestion of silica particles leads to the destruction of the lung macrophages. The destruction of macrophages accounts for an increased susceptibility to tuberculosis in persons with silicosis. Again, people with acute silicosis appear to be at considerably higher risk of developing tuberculosis. "Egg shell" calcification of hilar lymph nodes also can occur in silicosis.

7. **What is "shrinking lungs" syndrome?**

   It is estimated that weakness of the diaphragm and other respiratory muscles is found in about 25% of patients with SLE. This accounts for the previously unexplained findings of dyspnea without evidence of interstitial or pulmonary vascular disease. These patients have subsegmental atelectasis, an elevated diaphragm on chest radiograph, and restrictive physiology. This has been referred to as the unexplained dyspnea and shrinking lungs syndrome (*Ref: Fishman's Pulmonary Diseases and Disorders, 4th edition, Pg 1201*).

8. What is Caplan's syndrome?

Caplan's syndrome refers to a radiographic picture that developed in Welsh coal miners who have coexistent coal worker's pneumoconiosis and rheumatoid arthritis. It consists of the sudden appearance of discrete nodules primarily in the upper lobes that are histologically identical to the necrobiotic (rheumatoid) nodule.

9. What is the sensitivity of various immunological tests associated with rheumatic disorders that may cause interstitial lung disease?

The sensitivity of commonly available immunological tests to diagnose the various rheumatic disorders associated with interstitial lung disease are as follows (Table 5.2) (*Ref: Fishman's Pulmonary Diseases and Disorders, 4th edition, Pg 1112*).

Table 5.2: Various immunological tests associated with rheumatic disorders

Rheumatic disorder	Sensitivity of test
Rheumatoid arthritis	Rheumatoid factor—72 to 85%
SLE	ds DNA—60 to 70%
Drug LE	ss DNA—80%
Sjögren's syndrome	Anti Ro—8 to 70%
Scleroderma	Anti Scl 70—15 to 50%
Polymyositis	Anti Jo 1—20 to 50%
Wegener's granulomatosis	c ANCA—75 to 95%
Churg-Strauss syndrome	c ANCA—80%
Goodpasture's syndrome	p ANCA–10 to 38%

The routine tests that should be ordered in all patients in whom interstitial lung disease is suspected include a complete and differential blood count, a blood chemistry panel including calcium, liver function tests, and a urinalysis.

10. **What is meant by "PIE" syndrome?**

    "PIE' syndrome or pulmonary infiltrates with eosinophilia include distinct individual syndromes characterized by eosinophilic pulmonary infiltrates (usually fleeting or migrating infiltrates) and peripheral blood eosinophilia. Eosinophilia is the presence of more than 500 eosinophils per microliter of blood. The common causes of "PIE" syndromes are the following:
    - Parasitic infestations—filariasis, strongyloides, etc.
    - Allergic bronchopulmonary mycoses
    - Vasculitic disorders—Churg-Strauss syndrome
    - Acute eosinophilic pneumonia
    - Chronic eosinophilic pneumonia
    - Eosinophilia—myalgia syndrome
    - Hypereosinophilic syndrome
    - Loffler's syndrome or simple pulmonary eosinophilia
    - Drugs—nitrofurantoin, sulfonamides, thiazides, etc.

    "PIE" syndromes are clinically characterized by the presence of low grade fever, nonproductive cough, dyspnea (mild to severe) wheezing and occasional hemoptysis. In general, glucocorticoids are the main stay of therapy in all the above mentioned conditions. PIE syndrome due to filarial infection is otherwise known as tropical pulmonary eosinophilia (TPE).

11. **What is hypersensitivity pneumonitis?**

    Hypersensitivity pneumonitis (HP), or extrinsic allergic alveolitis, is a spectrum of interstitial, alveolar, and bronchiolar lung diseases resulting from immunologically induced inflammation in response to inhalation of a wide variety of different materials that are usually organic. This inflammation ultimately leads to irreversible damage of the lungs. Some common agents that are associated with hypersensitivity pneumonitis include the following:

- Thermophilic actinomycetes cause Farmer's lung disease
- Aspergillus clavatus cause Malt worker's lung
- Bird proteins cause Bird fancier's lung.

Despite the terms "hypersensitivity" and "allergic", HP is not an atopic disease and is not associated with increased IgE levels or eosinophils (unlike the PIE syndromes). The clinical presentation may be acute or chronic. The chronic form of the disease clinically mimics idiopathic pulmonary fibrosis (i.e. gradual onset of dyspnea, dry cough and weight loss without fever).

Chapter 6

Tuberculosis

1. **What is latent tuberculosis?**

   In persons with intact cell mediated immunity, the primary infection with the tubercle bacilli is contained within granulomas in the lung parenchyma. This parenchymal tuberculous granuloma is called as the Ghon focus (usually in the right upper lobe). From here, the tubercle bacilli then drain to the regional lymph nodes. These lymph nodes also often caseate. This combination of caseated parenchymal lung lesion and regional lymph node is referred to as the Ghon complex or primary complex. This primary infection may be asymptomatic. These granuloma later on calcify. The calcified primary parenchymal lung lesion or the calcified primary parenchymal lesion plus the calcified hilar lymph node (i.e. the Ranke complex) may be seen radiologically. These calcified lesions on the chest X-ray are evidences of healed primary tuberculosis (Fig. 6.1).

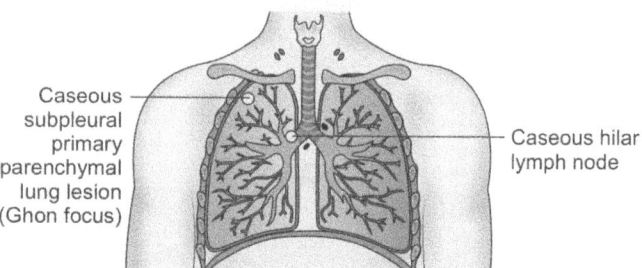

Fig. 6.1: Primary tuberculous infection

> **Ghon focus + Caseous hilar lymph node = Ghon complex**
>
> **Calcified Ghon focus + Calcified hilar lymph node = Ranke complex**

However, some viable tubercle bacilli may lie dormant within these granulomas for years. Such a person is said to be infected with tuberculosis, but he does not have active disease. This stage is called as the latent tuberculosis infection (LTBI). Reactivation of the primary disease may occur in such a person if his immune status is compromised. Newer techniques for the diagnosis of latent infection include the QuantiFERON-TB and the T SPOT-TB test. These immunological tests are based on the detection of interferon gamma produced by T cells exposed to *Mycobacterium tuberculosis*. These tests are more sensitive and more specific in immunosuppressed patients.

2. What is the natural history of primary or Ghon's complex?

In majority of the cases, where the immune response of the person enables the primary complex to contain the tuberculous infection, these lesions become fibrotic and may subsequently become calcified. In a minority of infected cases, the primary complex give rise to overt progressive primary tuberculosis which may manifest in a number of ways as follows (Boxes 6.1 and 6.2, and Fig. 6.2):

Box 6.1: Complications arising from the primary parenchymal lesion or Ghon focus

- Rupture into the pleural space resulting in pleural effusion
- Rupture into the bronchus resulting in tuberculous bronchopneumonia
- Enlargement of the focus to form a circular coin lesion. The circular coin lesion may heal with calcification or it may progress to a characteristic post-primary lesion containing abundant caseous necrotic tissue called as the tuberculoma
- Hematogenous dissemination of the bacilli from the focus can cause fatal non-pulmonary disease involving the central nervous system, bones, kidneys or miliary tuberculosis

Box 6.2: Complications arising from the involved mediastinal lymph node

- Bronchial obstruction causing collapse of the lung lobes
- Rupture of the node into the pericardium causes pericardial effusion

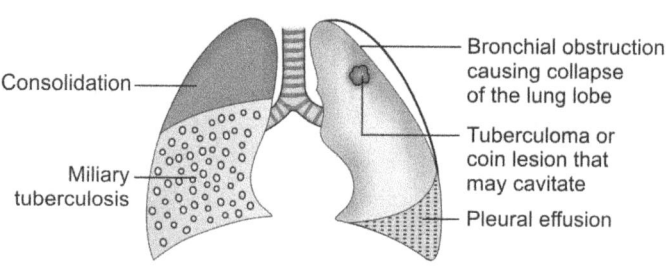

Fig. 6.2: Complications of primary tuberculosis

3. **What are the features that indicate active post-primary pulmonary tuberculosis?**

   Post-primary tuberculosis refers to exogenous (i.e. newly acquired) or endogenous (i.e. reactivation of a dormant primary lesion) infection in a person who has been sensitized by earlier exposure to tubercle bacilli. Features suggesting active post primary pulmonary tuberculosis include the following (Box 6.3) (*Ref: The Washington Manual of Medical Therapeutics, 33rd edition*).

> **Box 6.3:** Features suggesting reactivation of pulmonary tuberculosis
>
> - Pulmonary symptoms like cough with expectoration, hemoptysis, etc.
> - Presence of systemic symptoms like fever, tiredness, anorexia and unexplained significant weight loss (>5% weight loss in 1 month or >10% weight loss in 6 months)
> - Presence of coarse crackles on auscultation
> - Demonstration of acid-fast bacilli in the sputum or early morning gastric washings or bronchoalveolar lavage fluid by microscopy (Ziehl-Neelsen staining), culture or molecular DNA technology (PCR)
> - Raised ESR, CRP and a positive PPD skin test (induration ≥ 5 mm)
> - Radiological features like presence of cavities, ill-defined soft or cloudy shadows and rapid progression of these shadows on serial X-rays

4. What is the significance of a positive PPD skin test?

A positive PPD tuberculin skin test is an example of a delayed hypersensitivity reaction. The test can be positive within 3 to 8 weeks after exposure to *Mycobacterium tuberculosis*. A positive PPD skin test indicates only infection with *mycobacteria* and not active disease. Active disease should be confirmed by the growth of *Mycobacterium tuberculosis* in respiratory secretions or other body fluids or tissues.

The PPD skin test is usually done by the Mantoux method (i.e. measurement of the diameter of induration of skin after 48–72 hours of intradermal injection of 0.1 mL (5 TU) of tuberculin protein). The PPD skin test is negative in about 25% of patients with active tuberculosis (Figs 6.3 and 6.4).

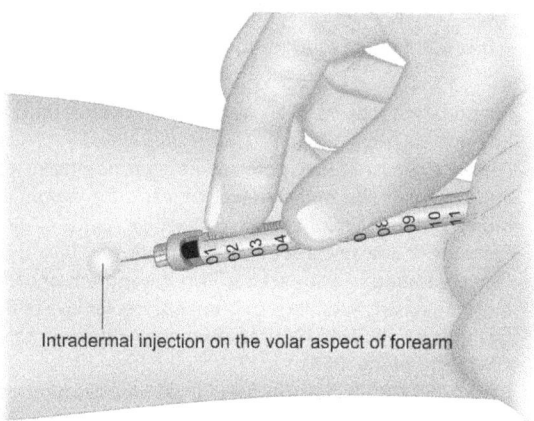

Fig. 6.3: Administering intradermal tuberculin protein

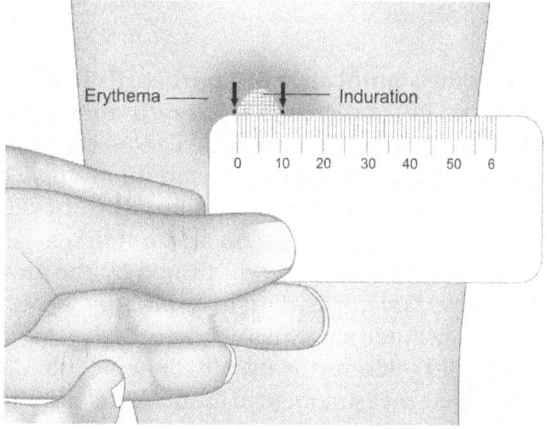

Fig. 6.4: Measuring the zone of induration across the forearm

5. What are the reasons for false-negative PPD skin test?

The PPD skin test is negative in about 25% of patients with active tuberculosis. A false-negative PPD result is seen in the following circumstances (Box 6.4):

> **Box 6.4:** False-negative PPD skin test
> - Recent viral infections, HIV infection
> - Those with chronic renal failure, leukemia, lymphoma etc.
> - Those with extreme malnutrition
> - Corticosteroid and other immunosuppressive drug therapy, recent live virus vaccinations, etc.
> - Miliary tuberculosis
> - Sarcoidosis
> - Extremes of age, i.e. newborns and elderly patients

6. What do you know about the specificity of PPD skin test?

The specificity of a positive PPD reaction is variable and is dependent on the prevalence of infection with non-tuberculous mycobacteria in that particular region. The PPD test may be falsely positive in those who had prior BCG vaccination and in areas where the exposure to non-tuberculous mycobacteria is high.

If the PPD skin test is strongly positive (i.e. more than 15 mm induration), and no other diagnosis is established, then empirical antituberculosis treatment (ATT) should be initiated in a sputum smear negative and culture awaited patient with suspected tuberculosis. If there is a favorable clinical or radiographic response within 3 months of initiation of the empirical therapy, then the empirical treatment should be continued. If there is no favorable response during this period, then the empirical treatment should be discontinued (*Ref: Fishman's, 4th edition, Pg 2483*).

7. What are the peculiarities of tuberculosis in the elderly?

There are some special features in the clinical presentation of tuberculosis in the elderly people. These are the following:
- Symptoms may be atypical (fever, sweating, hemoptysis may be absent)
- Hepatosplenomegaly (25–50% of cases)
- PPD skin test may be negative
- Sputum smears may be negative (hence sputum culture is important)
- Atypical chest X-ray features (bi-basal pneumonia, absent cavitation, etc.).

Thus in elderly, a cryptic presentation, i.e. fever of unknown origin often accompanied by pancytopenia or leukemoid reaction, is a common mode of presentation. The disseminated lung lesions are usually too small to be visible on the chest X-ray which is often deceptively normal. Hence, this variant is called as cryptic disseminated tuberculosis.

8. What is the management protocol for ATT induced hepatotoxicity?

If the liver function tests are deranged, then hold all the hepatotoxic antituberculous drugs until the symptoms resolve and the transaminases decrease to less than two times of their normal values. A nonhepatotoxic regimen consisting of ethambutol, fluoroquinolone and streptomycin should be started if treatment cannot be withheld due to the patient's clinical condition. Once the transaminases have decreased to less than two times of their normal values and the hepatotoxic symptoms of the patient have resolved, then we can rechallenge the patient by adding drugs one by one to the regimen every 4th day as shown below.

- **R**ifampin (10 mg/kg/day) for 3 days—if patient is asymptomatic, then add
- **I**NH (5 mg/kg/day) for 3 days—if patient is asymptomatic, then add
- **P**yrazinamide (15-25 mg/kg/day).

If signs and symptoms of hepatitis recur with rechallenge, then discontinue the responsible drug and modify the antituberculous regimen.

9. What are the antituberculous regimens that can be used in patients with chronic liver disease?

In patients with advanced liver disease, liver function tests should be done at the start of treatment. The more unstable or severe the liver disease is, the fewer hepatotoxic drugs should be used. If the serum alanine aminotransferase level is more than 3 times normal before the initiation of treatment, then the following regimen is considered to be the most ideal:

- 18-24 months of Streptomycin plus Ethambutol plus a Fluoroquinolone

Clinical and biochemical monitoring (liver function tests) of all patients with pre-existing liver disease should be performed regularly during treatment.

10. What is the difference between MDR tuberculosis and XDR tuberculosis?

Multiple drug resistant tuberculosis (MDR-TB) is defined as resistance to at least both isoniazid and rifampin. Extensively drug resistant tuberculosis (XDR-TB) is defined as resistance to isoniazid and rifampin plus resistance to any fluoroquinolone and at least one of the three injectable second-line drugs (amikacin, kanamycin, capreomycin, etc.).

11. What is the role of "DOTS" and "DOTS–Plus" in the treatment of tuberculosis?

"DOTS" stands for "**D**irectly **O**bserved **T**reatment, **S**hort-course" and is a major plank in the WHO global initiative to stop tuberculosis. The DOTS strategy focuses on five main targets of action. These include the following:

- Government commitment to control TB
- Diagnosis based on sputum-smear microscopy tests done on patients who actively report symptoms suggestive of tuberculosis
- Direct observation short-course chemotherapy treatments (thrice weekly regimens)
- A definite supply of drugs
- Standardized reporting and recording of cases and treatment outcomes.

The WHO extended the DOTS program in 1998 to include the treatment of MDR-TB. This is the "DOTS-Plus" program.

12. How will you manage tuberculosis in pregnant and lactating patients?

A pregnant woman should be advised that successful treatment of tuberculosis with the standard regimen is important for the successful outcome of pregnancy. With the exception of streptomycin, all the first line antituberculous drugs are safe for use in pregnancy. Streptomycin is **ototoxic** to the fetus and should not be used during pregnancy.

A breastfeeding woman who has tuberculosis should receive the full course of antituberculous treatment. Timely and properly applied chemotherapy is the best way to prevent transmission of tubercle bacilli to the baby. Mother and baby should stay together and the baby should continue to breastfeed. After active tuberculosis in the baby has been ruled out, the baby should be given 6 months of isoniazid preventive therapy (chemoprophylaxis), followed by Bacillus Calmette-Guérin (BCG) vaccination.

13. What is extrapulmonary tuberculosis?

Extrapulmonary tuberculosis (EPTB) refers to a case of tuberculosis involving organs other than the lung parenchyma, e.g. pleura, lymph nodes, abdomen, genitourinary tract, skin, joints, bones or meninges. Mycobacterial infection involving the cervical lymph nodes (i.e. scrofula) is the most common form of extra-pulmonary tuberculosis. The most common site for tuberculosis infection of the bone is the thoracic spine. Most often, the lesion in the spine is paradiscal in location with destruction of the disc, reduction of the disc space and concomitant destruction of the vertebral bodies.

(**Note:** Miliary tuberculosis is classified as pulmonary tuberculosis because of the presence of lesions in the lung parenchyma).

14. How will you manage a case of extrapulmonary tuberculosis?

Both pulmonary and extrapulmonary tuberculosis should be treated with the same regimen (2HRZE / 4HR). In tuberculous meningitis, ethambutol should be replaced with streptomycin. This is because streptomycin readily penetrates the inflamed meninges and enters into the cerebrospinal fluid (CSF). Experts recommend 12 months of treatment for tuberculous meningitis because of the serious risk of disability and mortality associated with meningitis. For tuberculosis of the bones or joints, 9 months of treatment is recommended because of the difficulties in assessing treatment response in those conditions. Adjuvant corticosteroid treatment (during the initial 6-8 weeks) is recommended only for tuberculous meningitis, tuberculous pericarditis and severe miliary tuberculosis.

15. How do you interpret ESR and CRP values in day to day practice?

The erythrocyte sedimentation rate (ESR) is a composite measure of plasma protein composition, concentration and erythrocyte morphology. The most common cause of an increased ESR is an acute phase response, which causes an increase in plasma protein concentration. Such acute phase responses occur in the setting of acute or chronic bacterial, fungal or viral infections.

However, some conditions which increase plasma protein composition and concentration without creating an acute phase response (multiple myeloma, end stage renal disease, old age, pregnancy, connective tissue diseases, etc.) are also associated with raised ESR. The normal range of ESR in adult males is less than 10 mm/hr and that in females is less than 20 mm/hr. The ESR value usually rises with age. The upper limit of normal range of ESR for an adult can be calculated as follows (*Ref: Oxford Handbook of Clinical Medicine*).

$$\text{Males} = \frac{\text{Age in years}}{2} \quad \text{Females} = \frac{\text{Age in years} + 10}{2}$$

C-reactive protein (CRP) is an acute phase reactant synthesized by the liver usually in response to active inflammation triggered by organisms like bacteria or fungi. CRP opsonises the invading pathogens. So, the levels of CRP are raised in the setting of bacterial, fungal or viral infections. But CRP levels are not influenced by plasma protein composition and concentration. Hence, diseases which alter plasma protein concentration **without** creating an acute phase response do not affect the CRP value. Hence, the simultaneous estimation of both ESR and CRP values would help to narrow down the differential diagnosis. The normal CRP value is less than 10 mg/L.

16. How do you confirm the diagnosis of active pulmonary tuberculosis?

A confident diagnosis of active tuberculosis requires bacteriologic confirmation. It is important to remember that a positive acid-fast smear is not specific for M. tuberculosis (saprophytic mycobacteria are also acid-fast). Hence, sputum culture is the only absolute way of confirming the diagnosis.

If the patient is not spontaneously producing sputum, induced sputum can be obtained by nebulising the patient with isotonic or hypertonic saline for 5 to 15 minutes. In some cases, bronchoscopy may be considered to obtain the sputum sample. Sputum culture for acid-fast bacilli (AFB) is ideally done in the liquid medium (i.e. BACTEC or MGIT) for rapid results (within 7–21 days).

17. What is "open-negative" syndrome?

There is an entity called as "open-negative syndrome" in post-primary pulmonary tuberculosis. It consists of thin walled, innocuous, epithelized inactive cavities. It is seen in properly treated cases of tuberculosis. These cavities are also referred to as " INH cavities". Although these cavities themselves will not produce any symptoms, they are associated with certain hazards like secondary bacterial infection, spontaneous pneumothorax, colonization with fungi, etc.

18. What are the differences in the characteristics of post-primary tuberculosis in non-immunosuppressed and immunosuppressed persons?

The important differences in the characteristics of post-primary tuberculosis in non-immunosuppressed and immunosuppressed persons are the following (Table 6.1):

Table 6.1: Differences in the characteristics of post-primary tuberculosis in non-immunosuppressed and immunosuppressed persons

Characteristics	Non-immunosuppressed	Immuno-suppressed
Pulmonary cavitation	Prominent	Absent
Localization by fibrosis	Marked	Limited
Intrathoracic lymphadenopathy	Uncommon	Common
Miliary disease	Uncommon	Common
Atelectasis	Uncommon	Common
Lymphatic and hematogenous dissemination	Uncommon	Common
Empyema	Uncommon	Common
Tuberculin test	Positive	Negative
Adverse drug reactions	Uncommon	Common
Relapse following therapy	Uncommon	Common

19. What is a Rasmussen aneurysm?

A Rasmussen aneurysm is a pseudoaneurysm of a pulmonary artery caused by erosion from an adjacent tuberculous cavity. These pseudoaneurysms are uncommon and may form months to years after formation of the cavity. Hemoptysis is the usual presenting symptom, which may be massive and life threatening.

20. What is meant by broncholithiasis?
Broncholithiasis is an uncommon complication of pulmonary tuberculosis that is caused by calcified peribronchial nodes. These nodes either erode into or cause considerable distortion of an adjacent bronchus. Although any bronchus may be involved, a right-sided predominance has been observed. The right middle lobe is served by an unusually long and thin bronchus that is particularly prone to obstruction. Presenting symptoms may include cough, hemoptysis, wheezing, or evidence of recurrent pneumonia.

21. What is middle lobe or Brock's syndrome?
Middle lobe syndrome is defined as recurrent or chronic collapse of the middle lobe of the right lung. It occurs in all age groups and is divided into an obstructive type, with a demonstrable airway occlusion, and a nonobstructive type, with a patent right middle lobe bronchus apparent on bronchoscopy. The reported etiologies of the middle lobe syndrome are the following:
- Inflammation (47%)
- Malignant tumors (22%)
- Bronchiectasis (15%)
- Tuberculosis (9%)
- Benign tumors (2%)
- Aspiration (2%)

The propensity of the right middle lobe to collapse is explained by its anatomical peculiarities which include the following:
- The origin of the right middle lobe bronchus is often narrow and so it is easily obstructed

- The middle lobe bronchus is surrounded by lymph nodes whose enlargement by inflammation or tumor may cause extrinsic compression
- The middle lobe is separated from the right upper and lower lobes by fissures, and therefore has poor collateral ventilation from the surrounding areas.

22. Which are the diseases associated with granuloma formation in the lung?

A granuloma is a focal, compact collection of inflammatory cells. The predominating cells are the mononuclear cells (i.e. macrophages and T lymphocytes). It is usually formed as a result of the persistence of a non-degradable product of active hypersensitivity in the body. Some important diseases associated with granuloma formation in the lungs are the following (Box 6.5):

> **Box 6.5:** Granulomatous pulmonary diseases
>
> - Fungal infections
> - Mycobacterial infections
> - Wegener's granulomatosis
> - Churg-Strauss syndrome
> - Sarcoidosis
> - Hypersensitivity pneumonitis
> - Berylliosis
> - Silicosis

Chapter
7
Bronchiectasis

1. **What is bronchiectasis?**
   Bronchiectasis is defined as an abnormal and permanent dilatation of the cartilage containing airways. Bronchiectasis is more common in women and it usually affects the lower lobe bronchi. The left side is involved more frequently than the right side. Bronchiectasis results from the occurrence of one of the following three main pathogenic mechanisms:
   - Bronchial wall injury
   - Bronchial lumen obstruction
   - Traction from adjacent fibrosis

   The "vicious cycle hypothesis" proposed that an initial airway insult (such as an infection), often on the background of genetic susceptibility and compromised host clearance mechanisms (in particular, the mucociliary mechanism), facilitated persistent bacterial colonization and infection. This initiates a secondary host inflammatory response. This in turn causes further damage to the airway wall. The predominant symptoms are chronic productive cough with copious sputum (early morning cough) and hemoptysis. The principal clinical sign is coarse leathery crackles on auscultation of the chest.

2. **What do you know about the etiology and distribution of bronchiectatic changes in the lungs?**
   Bronchiectatic changes can affect any part of the lung depending upon the factor responsible for creating the airway insult (Table 7.1).

Table 7.1: Distribution of bronchiectatic changes in the lungs

Part of the lung affected	Most likely etiology
Lower lobes	• Interstitial lung disease • Chronic pulmonary infections *(usually bacterial)*
Right middle lobe	Obstruction by peribronchial nodes
Upper lobes	• Tuberculosis • Chronic fungal infections • ABPA *(central bronchi)*

3. What is dry bronchiectasis?

Dry bronchiectasis or bronchiectasis sicca is a type of traction bronchiectasis that predominantly affect the upper lobe. Traction bronchiectasis is seen in the setting of extensive lung fibrosis. The fibrosed parts of the lung pulls apart the surrounding airways, resulting in their dilatation. It usually occurs as post-tuberculous sequalae. It is more common on the right side. Since dry bronchiectasis is not associated with recurrent airway infection or obstruction, these patients usually present with episodes of marked hemoptysis without sputum production.

4. Which are the syndromes usually associated with bronchiectasis?

A number of syndromes and clinical conditions are associated with bronchiectasis and they include the following (Box 7.1):

Box 7.1: Conditions associated with bronchiectasis

- Primary ciliary dyskinesia—approximately 50% of patients with this condition have Kartagener's syndrome which is a triad of situs inversus, sinusitis and bronchiectasis

Contd...

Contd...

> - Yellow nail syndrome—triad of yellow-green discoloration of the nails, lymphedema of the lower extremities and lymphocyte predominant pleural effusion
> - Young's syndrome—combination of obstructive azoospermia (with normal spermatogenesis) and chronic sinopulmonary infections
> - Bruton agammaglobulinemia
> - Allergic bronchopulmonary aspergillosis (ABPA)
> - Right middle lobe syndrome (Brock's syndrome): Recurrent atelectasis associated with bronchiectasis of the right middle lobe. It is commonly seen in tuberculosis. The right middle lobe is commonly affected because the right middle lobe bronchus is surrounded by a chain of lymph nodes at its origin and it gets compressed easily

5. What are the important complications of bronchiectasis?

Bronchiectasis is a chronic inflammatory condition. The important complications of bronchiectasis are the following (Box 7.2):

> **Box 7.2:** Complications of bronchiectasis
>
> - Hemoptysis
> - Recurrent pneumonia
> - Lung abscess
> - Empyema
> - Metastatic abscesses
> - Purulent pericarditis
> - Cor pulmonale
> - Hypoproteinemia
> - Secondary amyloidosis

Bronchiectasis is not a premalignant condition. *Haemophilus influenzae* is the most common organism recovered from non-cystic fibrosis patients with bronchiectasis (*Ref: CMDT 2014*). Hypoproteinemia occurs due to the loss of albumin in sputum. Splenomegaly can occur in some cases of bronchi-ectasis with secondary amyloidosis.

6. What is pseudobronchiectasis?

Bronchiectatic changes seen in certain conditions like chronic bronchitis, acute pneumonia and allergic bronchopulmonary aspergillosis are reversible. So, this type of bronchiectasis is sometimes referred to as pseudobronchiectasis.

7. What do you know about cystic fibrosis?

Cystic fibrosis is a cause of severe chronic lung disease in young adults. It is an autosomal recessive disorder. Cystic fibrosis is caused by abnormalities in a membrane chloride channel [the cystic fibrosis transmembrane conductance regulator (CFTR) protein] that results in altered chloride transport and water flux across the apical surface of epithelial cells. So in people with cystic fibrosis, almost all exocrine glands produce an abnormal mucus that obstructs glands and ducts and leads to tissue damage.

In the respiratory tract, inadequate hydration of the tracheobronchial epithelium impairs mucociliary function. High concentration of DNA in airway secretions (due to chronic airway inflammation and autolysis of neutrophils) increases the sputum viscosity, resulting in a variety of pulmonary manifestations including bronchiectasis and atelectasis.

8. What are the important respiratory complications of cystic fibrosis?

The lungs are macroscopically normal at birth, but bronchiolar inflammation and infections usually lead to bronchiectasis in childhood. At this stage, the lungs are most commonly infected with *Staphylococcus aureus*. However, in adulthood, many patients with cystic fibrosis become chronically colonized with *Pseudomonas aeruginosa*. The important respiratory complications of cystic fibrosis are the following (Box 7.3):

> **Box 7.3:** Complications of cystic fibrosis
>
> - Infective exacerbations of bronchiectasis
> - Spontaneous pneumothorax
> - Hemoptysis
> - Nasal polyps
> - Cor pulmonale
> - Respiratory failure
> - Lobar collapse due to thick secretions

9. **What is the definitive treatment for cystic fibrosis?**
    Lung transplantation is currently the only definitive treatment for advanced cystic fibrosis. Double lung or heart-lung transplantation is required.
    Ivacaftor is a new oral drug, available for the 5% of cystic fibrosis patients with a G551D mutation. Ivacaftor is a potentiator of the CFTR channel that works by increasing the time the channel remains open after being activated.

10. **What are the important diagnostic features of allergic bronchopulmonary aspergillosis (ABPA)?**
    Allergic bronchopulmonary aspergillosis is caused by a hypersensitivity reaction to the fungus *Aspergillus fumigatus*. ABPA may develop in 10% of patients with cystic fibrosis. Patients with ABPA may display the following diagnostic criteria proposed by Greenberger and Patterson (Box 7.4).

> **Box 7.4:** Criteria for diagnosis of ABPA
>
> - History of asthma
> - Elevated total IgE (>1,000 IU/mL)
> - Elevated serum anti-AF IgE and IgG
> - Positive immediate hypersensitivity skin test to aspergillus
> - Serum precipitins to aspergillus fumigatus

Radiologically, these patients may have patchy, fleeting infiltrates on the chest X-ray. HRCT may show central bronchiectasis. It should be remembered that the presence of *Aspergillus fumigatus* in sputum is only a minor criterion for the diagnosis of ABPA. The treatment consists of long-term systemic corticosteroids (oral prednisolone 7.5–10 mg daily).

11. **What are the imaging studies that can be done in a case of bronchiectasis?**

    Radiographic abnormalities include dilated and thickened bronchi that may appear as "tram-tracks" or as ring-like markings on chest radiograph. Scattered irregular opacities, atelectasis, and focal consolidation may also be present. High-resolution CT scan (HRCT) is the diagnostic study of choice in bronchiectasis (Fig. 7.1).

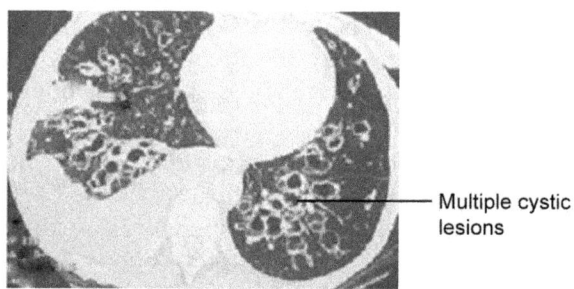

Fig. 7.1: HRCT in bronchiectasis

Chapter 8

Pneumonia

1. **How do you classify pneumonia?**
   Pneumonia is defined as a potentially fatal infection and inflammation of the lower respiratory tract (i.e. bronchioles and alveoli). It is usually caused by inhaled bacteria. Based on the anatomical part of the lung parenchyma involved, pneumonia is traditionally classified into the following three types (Fig. 8.1):
   a. **Lobar pneumonia:** Occurs due to acute bacterial infection of part of a lobe or complete lobe. Whole lobe is often affected as the inflammation spreads through the pores of Khon and Lambert channels.
   b. **Bronchopneumonia:** Acute bacterial infection of the terminal bronchioles characterized by purulent exudates which extends into surrounding alveoli through endobronchial route resulting in patchy consolidation. It is usually seen in extremes of age and also in association with chronic debilitating conditions.
   c. **Interstitial pneumonia:** Patchy inflammatory changes, caused by viral or mycoplasma infection, mostly confined to the interstitial tissue of the lung without alveolar exudates. It is characterized by alveolar septal edema and mononuclear infiltrates.

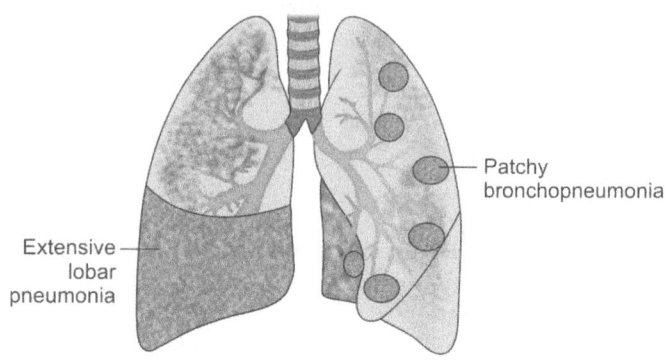

Fig. 8.1: Types of pneumonia

Clinically, it is ideal to classify pneumonia according to the setting in which it occurs. This helps the treating physician to give the appropriate empirical antimicrobial therapy. Accordingly pneumonia may be classified as community acquired pneumonia or CAP (typical and atypical CAP), nosocomial pneumonia, aspiration pneumonia, pneumonia in immune-compromised host and necrotizing pneumonia.

2. **What is community-acquired pneumonia or CAP?**
Community-acquired pneumonia or CAP is defined as "an acute infection of the pulmonary parenchyma that is associated with at least some symptoms of acute infection, accompanied by the presence of an acute infiltrate on a chest radiograph or auscultatory findings consistent with pneumonia, in a patient not hospitalized for more than 14 days before the onset of symptoms." *Streptococcus pneumoniae* is the most common etiologic agent of CAP.

3. What is hospital-acquired pneumonia or HAP?

Hospital acquired pneumonia or HAP is defined as pneumonia that occurs 48 hours or more after admission to a hospital or health care facility. HAP is usually caused by bacteria. About 60% of the cases of nosocomial pneumonia are caused by aerobic gram-negative bacilli like *Pseudomonas*, 20% by *Staphylococcus aureus* (including MRSA), 10% by *Staphylococcus pneumoniae* and the rest by anaerobes.

4. What is CURB-65 score?

Community-acquired pneumonia (CAP) is usually spread by droplet infection and most of the cases occur in previously healthy individuals. CURB-65 score is a severity assessment scale used to determine the management protocol of CAP. It includes the following parameters (Fig. 8.2).

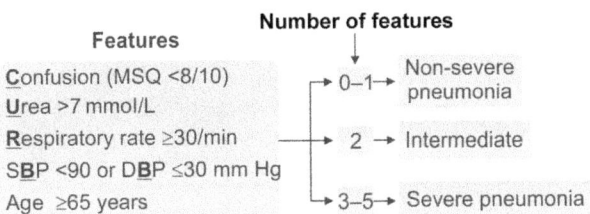

Fig. 8.2: CURB score calculation

A patient with a score of 3 or more is considered as having severe pneumonia and has to be managed in a hospital. He should be immediately started on empirical antibiotic therapy. The preferred antibiotic regimen is parentral ceftriaxone plus clarithromycin (*Ref: Washington Manual, 33rd edition*).

5. What are the different pathological and clinical stages seen in lobar pneumonia?

The classic clinical features of consolidation are seen in lobar pneumonia. In lobar pneumonia, part of a lobe, a whole lobe or more than one lobe (called massive consolidation) may be involved. The various stages are as follows. Initially there is the pathological stage of congestion which lasts for about 2 days. The early inflammatory response produces features like fever, cough with expectoration, and indux crackles are audible on auscultation during this stage (Fig. 8.3).

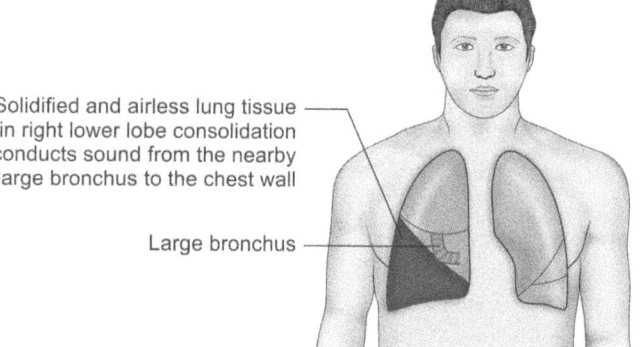

Fig. 8.3: Consolidated and airless lung in lobar pneumonia conducts tubular bronchial breath sounds from nearby large bronchi directly to the chest wall without filtration

During the next 6–8 days, the involved areas of the lung go through the pathological stages of red and gray hepatization. The diseased lung tissue is dry, airless and solidified. So in addition to the earlier clinical features, tubular bronchial breath sounds are heard on auscultation of the chest wall. Thus, the classic clinical signs of "consolidation" are present during these stages. In some cases, there is synpneumonic pleural effusion associated with consolidation. In these patients, the clinical signs of consolidation will be masked by those of pleural effusion.

This is followed by the stage of resolution with redux crackles, and this stage lasts for 1–4 weeks. In this era of early antibiotic therapy, the stage of resolution usually directly follows the stage of congestion, without going through the stages of red and gray hepatization. Hence, the classical clinical signs of consolidation may not be present in many cases of pneumonia. Also, it should be remembered that radiographic changes resolve slowly and lag behind clinical recovery. It takes about 4 weeks for the complete resolution of radiographic changes (radiological clearance is faster for atypical pathogens).

6. **What is meant by "consolidation" in pneumonia?**
During the stage of congestion, inflammatory cells invade the walls of the alveoli. The alveolar air spaces fill with a protein-rich exudative fluid. This is associated with significant hypoxemia because the thick inflammatory exudate interferes with the diffusion of oxygen and carbon dioxide. This alveolar exudate tends to solidify and this process is known as "consolidation".

7. **What are the causes for nonresolving pneumonia?**
Nonresolving pneumonia is defined as the persistence of radiographic abnormalities for a period of more than one month in a clinically improved host (*Ref: UpToDate Medicine*). The important causes are the following (Box 8.1):

> **Box 8.1:** Causes for nonresolving pneumonia
>
> - Inappropriate antibiotics
> - Resistant organisms
> - Immunosuppressed patient
> - Empyema formation
> - Bronchial obstruction due to any cause
> - Recurrent aspiration

A chest radiograph should be arranged after 6 weeks for all patients with pneumonia who are at higher risk of underlying malignancy (*smokers, those aged >50 years*) to rule out the possibility of nonresolving pneumonia.

8. **What are the features of "atypical" pneumonia?**

   "Atypical" pneumonia (*interstitial pneumonia*) accounts for about 60% of cases of community-acquired pneumonia. The common organisms responsible for causing "atypical" pneumonia are *Mycoplasma pneumonia*, viruses, *Chlamydia Pneumonia*, *Legionella pneumophila*, *Coxiella burnetti* and *Pneumocystis jirovecii*. The general features of atypical pneumonia include the following (Box 8.2):

> **Box 8.2:** Features of atypical pneumonia
>
> - Subacute onset of symptoms
> - Prominent constitutional symptoms like malaise, anorexia, etc.
> - Nonproductive cough and low to moderate grade fever
> - Lymphocytic inflammatory exudate mostly in the interstitium (eosinophilic alveolar exudate only in pneumocystis jirovecii pneumonia)
> - Chest X-ray shows diffuse interstitial pattern

The current guidelines recommend a macrolide antibiotic for the empirical treatment of atypical pneumonia. The fungus *Pneumocystis jirovecii* is an important pathogen that causes pneumonia in the immunocompromised host.

9. What are the important complications of pneumonia?

Prognosis in a case of pneumonia is generally good in an otherwise healthy patient with uncomplicated pneumonia. With appropriate treatment, most patients improve markedly within 2 weeks. Potential serious complications of pneumonia are multiple and include the following (Box 8.3):

> **Box 8.3:** Complications in pneumonia
>
> - Parapneumonic effusion (40% of patients)
> - Lung abscess and empyema
> - Retention of thick sputum causing lobar collapse
> - Pneumothorax: *Staphylococcus aureus, Pneumocystis jirovecii*
> - Ectopic abscess formation: Pneumocystis aureus
> - Immunological events, hemolytic anemia: *Mycoplasma pneumoniae*
> - Diarrhea, hyponatremia, encephalopathy: *Legionella pneumophila*
> - Hepatitis, pericarditis, myocarditis and meningoencephalitis
> - Acute respiratory distress syndrome (ARDS)

10. What is the role of aspiration in the etiology of lung abscess?

Lung abscess is a circumscribed area (>1 cm in diameter) of suppurative necrosis (pus) within the lung. Suppuration leading to lung abscess can result from primary, opportunistic or hematogenous lung infection. Bad orodental hygiene and other favorable conditions of aspiration like altered consciousness (due to alcohol, coma, etc.) are the important causative factors.

About 90% of primary lung abscess are caused by aspiration of oropharyngeal secretions. Aspiration abscesses are more common on the right side. In the supine position, the posterior segment of the right upper lobe or the apical segment of the right or left lower lobes are commonly involved. Lung abscess is usually caused by bacteria, particularly anaerobic bacilli (30–50% of cases), aerobic gram-positive cocci (25%) and aerobic gram-negative bacilli (5–12%). Polymicrobial infections are the most common type observed. Treatment include drainage (physiotherapy, postural or bronchoscopic), antibiotics for 4–6 weeks and surgical intervention, if medical therapy fails.

11. What is Mendelson's syndrome?

Aspiration of acidic gastric contents into the lungs can give rise to a severe hemorrhagic type of pneumonia which is often complicated by ARDS. This is referred to as the Mendelson's syndrome. This usually occurs in patients recovering from general anesthesia, due to poor gag reflex.

12. What is lipoid pneumonia?

Lipoid pneumonia is a chronic syndrome related to the repeated aspiration of oily materials, e.g. mineral oil, cod liver oil and oily nose drops. It usually occurs in elderly patients with impaired swallowing. Patchy opacities in dependent lung zones and lipid laden macrophages in expectorated sputum are characteristics of this condition.

13. Which are the clinical tools that help the clinician to narrow the differential diagnosis in a case of pneumonia occurring in an immunocompromised host?

Although almost any pathogen can cause pneumonia in an immunocompromised host. However three clinical tools help the clinician to narrow his differential diagnosis.

- **Knowledge of the underlying immunologic defect**: Specific immunologic defects are associated with particular infections. Defects in humoral immunity predispose to bacterial infections; defects in cellular immunity lead to infections with viruses, fungi, mycobacteria, and protozoa. Neutropenia and impaired granulocyte function predispose to infections from *Staphylococcus aureus*, *Aspergillus*, gram-negative bacilli and *Candida*.

- **The speed of onset of infection:** A fulminant pneumonia is often caused by bacterial infection, whereas an insidious pneumonia is more likely to be caused by viral, fungal, protozoal, or mycobacterial infection. w
- **The time course of infection:** Pneumonia occurring within 2–4 weeks after organ transplantation is usually bacterial, whereas pneumonia occurring several months or more after transplantation is more likely to be caused by *Pneumocystis jirovecii*, viruses (e.g. cytomegalovirus), and fungi (e.g. *Aspergillus*).

14. Which are the situations were rigid bronchoscopy is preferred over flexible bronchoscopy?

Rigid bronchoscopy is more advantageous in certain situations like evaluating massive hemoptysis and in removing foreign bodies. Endobronchial laser therapy and endobronchial stenting may be more easily performed with rigid bronchoscopy. Rigid bronchoscopy should be done only under general anesthesia.

Chapter 9

Diseases of the Airways and Lung Vasculature

1. What are the differentiating points between the two patterns of disease in advanced COPD?

Two classical phenotypes have been described among those suffering from chronic obstructive pulmonary disease (COPD), i.e. 'pink puffers' and 'blue bloaters'. The former are typically thin and breathless, and maintain a normal $PaCO_2$ until the late stage of disease. The latter develop hypercapnia earlier and may develop edema and secondary polycythemia. In practice, these two phenotypes often overlap (Table 9.1).

Table 9.1: Difference between pink puffer and blue bloater

	Type A: Pink puffer (Emphysema predominant)	Type B: Blue bloater (Bronchitis predominant)
History	• Major complaint is dyspnea, often severe, usually presenting after age 50 • Cough is rare, with only scant clear, mucoid sputum	• Main complaint is always chronic cough, productive of mucopurulent sputum, with frequent exacerbations due to chest infections • Often presents in late thirties • Dyspnea usually mild, though patients may note limitations to exercise capacity

Contd...

Contd...

Physical signs	• Patients are thin, with recent weight loss common • They appear uncomfortable, with evident use of accessory muscles of respiration • Chest is very quiet without any adventitious sound • No peripheral edema	• Patients frequently overweight and cyanotic • Comfortable at rest • Chest is noisy, with polyphonic wheezes • Peripheral edema is common
Laboratory studies	• Hemoglobin usually normal (12–15 g/dL) • PaO_2 normal to slightly reduced (65–75 mm Hg) • $PaCO_2$ normal to slightly reduced (35–40 mm Hg) • Chest radiograph shows hyperinflation with flattened diaphragms. Vascular markings are diminished, particularly at the apices	• Hemoglobin usually elevated (15–18 g/dL) • PaO_2 reduced (45–60 mm Hg) • $PaCO_2$ slightly to markedly elevated (50–60 mm Hg) • Chest radiograph usually shows increase in interstitial markings ("dirty lungs"), especially at bases. Diaphragms are not flattened
Pulmonary function test	• Total lung capacity increased • Diffusion capacity of CO is reduced • Static lung compliance increased	• Total lung capacity generally normal • Diffusion capacity of CO is normal • Static lung compliance normal

2. What is the role of steroids in the management of COPD?

Long-term use of inhaled steroids is recommended in the management of COPD in the following group of patients:

- In patients who experience two or more episodes of exacerbations per year. Exacerbations are defined as episodes of increased dyspnea and cough with change in the amount and character of sputum.
- In patients who demonstrate a significant amount of acute reversibility in response to inhaled anticholinergic or beta agonist bronchodilators.

The long-term use of oral steroids for the treatment of COPD is not recommended. Short course (i.e. 2 weeks) of oral steroids (30-40 mg of prednisolone) is recommended for the management of acute exacerbations of COPD. Their use has been proven to reduce the length of hospital stay, hasten recovery and reduce the chance of subsequent exacerbation or relapse. All forms of glucocorticosteroid therapy, even if inhaled or applied topically, can suppress the hypothalamic-pituitary-adrenal (HPA) axis. This is likely to result in a crisis due to adrenal insufficiency on withdrawal of the steroid in the following circumstances (*Ref: Davidson's Principles and Practice of Medicine, 20th edition*).

- If steroids have been administered for longer than **3 weeks**
- If the dose is higher than the **equivalent of 40 mg prednisolone** per day

> 5 mg prednisolone = 4 mg methylprednisolone = 20 mg hydrocortisone = 0.75 mg dexa/betamethasone

In these circumstances, the steroid drug, when it is no longer required for the underlying condition, must be withdrawn very slowly at a rate dictated by the duration of treatment. If the steroid therapy had been a prolonged one, then it may take many months for the HPA axis to recover.

3. **What are the causes for refractory asthma?**
   Inspite of maximal therapy, there is difficulty in controlling asthmatic symptoms in about 5% of patients. The common causes for refractory asthma are the following (Box 9.1):

   > **Box 9.1:** Causes for refractory asthma
   >
   > - Noncompliance with medication
   > - Exposure to high levels of allergens or unidentified occupational agents
   > - Associated severe rhinosinusitis or gastroesophageal reflux disease (GERD)
   > - Chronic infection with Mycoplasma or Chlamydia
   > - Concomitant use of drugs like beta-blockers, aspirin, etc.
   > - Associated diseases like hyper- or hypothyroidism

4. **What is intrinsic asthma?**
   Although majority of patients with asthma have atopy, in a proportion of patients with asthma there is no evidence of atopy or allergy. These patients have normal total and specific IgE levels. Skin tests are also negative. This type of nonatopic asthma is referred to as intrinsic asthma.

   This so called "intrinsic" asthma usually comes on later in life. It tends to be more severe than allergic asthma. The pathophysiology is very similar to that of allergic asthma and there is increasing evidence for local IgE production, possibly directed at bacterial or viral antigens.

5. **What are the important clinical differentiating features between asthma and COPD?**
   Slowly progressive respiratory symptoms in a middle-aged or elderly smoker are likely to indicate COPD.

However, such patients may also have asthma. Patients whose symptoms started before the age of 35 years are more likely to be asthmatic, particularly if they are nonsmokers with symptoms that vary in severity. The important clinical features that differentiate COPD from asthma are the following (Table 9.2):

Table 9.2: Features between COPD and asthma

Feature	COPD	Asthma
Smoking	Usually present	Not necessarily present
Age of onset of symptoms	More than 35 years	Less than 35 years
Chronic productive cough	Common	Uncommon
Breathlessness	Persistent and progressive	Variable
Night time waking up with breathlessness/wheeze	Uncommon	Common
Significant diurnal/day-to-day variability of symptoms	Uncommon	Common

6. What is the role of LTOT in the management of COPD?
GOLD stage 4 COPD patients (i.e. FEV_1/FVC <70% or FEV_1 <30% predicted) with very severe disease are benefitted by long-term domiciliary oxygen therapy or LTOT. LTOT has been shown to improve survival, prevent progression of pulmonary hypertension, decrease the incidence of secondary polycythemia and improve neuropsychological health. These patients should be instructed to use oxygen (2–4 liters/minute) for a minimum of 15 hours/day. The aim of the therapy is to increase the PaO_2 to at least 60 mm Hg.

7. What are the indications of noninvasive positive pressure ventilation or NIPPV in COPD?

An exacerbation of COPD is an event in the natural course of COPD characterized by an acute change in the patient's baseline dyspnea, cough and/or sputum production beyond the routine day-to-day variability that warrants a change in management strategy. Despite optimal pharmacologic management, severe cases of exacerbation of COPD necessitates ventilatory support, when the patient is unable to maintain his breathing function on his own. NIPPV is an option for patients who have respiratory failure and can no longer breathe on their own. The indications for NIPPV include the following (Box 9.2):

> **Box 9.2:** Indications for NIPPV or NIV
>
> - Severe hypercapnia (PaCO$_2$ >50 mm of Hg)
> - Severe respiratory acidosis (pH < 7.35)
> - Persistence of breathlessness even after optimal medical therapy

NIPPV provides ventilatory support to a patient through the upper airways. It enhances the breathing process by giving the patient a mixture of air and oxygen from a flow generator through a tightly fitted facial or nasal mask. It is also known as just noninvasive ventilation or NIV. NIV cannot be offered to very drowsy or non-cooperative patients. In such cases invasive mechanical ventilation may be required to support the respiration.

8. What do you know about the GOLD classification of COPD?

Global Initiative for Chronic Obstructive Lung Disease or GOLD guidelines have classified COPD into four stages depending upon the spirometric evaluation of the severity of airflow limitation. Spirometry should be performed after the administration of an adequate dose of a short acting inhaled bronchodilator in order to minimize variability. The GOLD classification is as follows (Fig. 9.1):

GOLD 1: Mild disease	$FEV_1 \geq 80\%$ predicted
GOLD 2: Moderate disease	$FEV_1 < 80\%$ predicted
GOLD 3: Severe disease	$FEV_1 < 50\%$ predicted
GOLD 4: Very severe disease	$FEV_1 < 30\%$ predicted

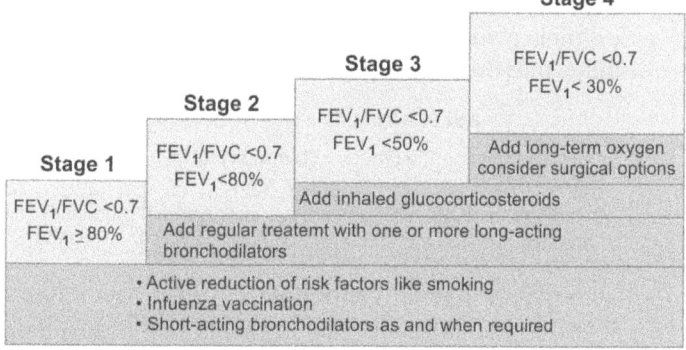

Fig. 9.1: GOLD classification of COPD (in patients with $FEV_1/FVC < 0.7$)

9. What is cor pulmonale?

The term cor pulmonale refers to the altered structure (hypertrophy/dilatation) and/or impaired function of the right ventricle that results from pulmonary hypertension that is associated with diseases of the lung, pulmonary vasculature, upper airway or chest wall. Cor pulmonale may be acute (e.g. in pulmonary thromboembolism); or chronic (e.g. severe COPD, obstructive sleep apnea, kyphoscoliosis, etc.). The different pathophysiological mechanisms that can lead to cor pulmonale are the following (Box 9.3):

> **Box 9.3:** Pathophysiological mechanisms of cor pulmonale
>
> - Pulmonary vasoconstriction (secondary to alveolar hypoxia)
> - Anatomic reduction of pulmonary vascular bed (emphysema, emboli, etc.)
> - Increased blood viscosity (polycythemia, sickle-cell disease, etc.)
> - Increased pulmonary blood flow (left-to-right shunts)

10. What is hepatopulmonary syndrome?

Hepatopulmonary syndrome is defined as a clinical disorder associated with advanced liver disease, pulmonary vascular dilatation and a defect in the oxygenation of blood, in the absence of detectable primary cardiopulmonary disease. The pulmonary vascular dilatations are caused by increased estrogen levels in the blood of patients with chronic liver disease (due to inability of the diseased liver to detoxify estrogen (Box 9.4)).

> **Box 9.4:** Features of hepatopulmonary syndrome
>
> - Advanced chronic liver disease
> - Absence of primary cardiopulmonary disease
> - Intrapulmonary vascular dilatation
> - Intrapulmonary arteriovenous shunting
> - Arterial hypoxemia

These vascular dilatations occur predominantly in the bases of the lung, and are sites of intrapulmonary arteriovenous shunting. Therefore, when the patient is sitting up, blood pools at the bases of the lung with resultant increased intrapulmonary arteriovenous shunting. This worsens the hypoxia and produces platypnea (shortness of breath relieved by lying down) and orthodeoxia (fall in the arterial PO_2 in the upright position). This hypoxia is responsible for the cyanosis and clubbing that occur in certain cases of chronic liver disease. Progressive and severe hypoxemia is an indication for liver transplantation and this is currently the only effective treatment for this condition.

11. **How does spirometry help to categorize between obstructive and restrictive ventilatory patterns?**

    Spirometry measures the rate at which the lung changes its volume during forced breathing maneuvers. The most important spirometric values that help to differentiate between obstructive and restrictive respiratory diseases are the FVC and FEV_1. The absolute FEV_1/FVC ratio distinguishes obstructive from restrictive spirometry patterns (Fig. 9.2).

    - FVC: Forced vital capacity, i.e. the total volume of air that can be exhaled after maximal inhalation during a forced expiratory effort.
    - FEV_1: Forced expiratory volume in one second, i.e. the volume of air exhaled forcefully in the first second after a maximal inhalation.

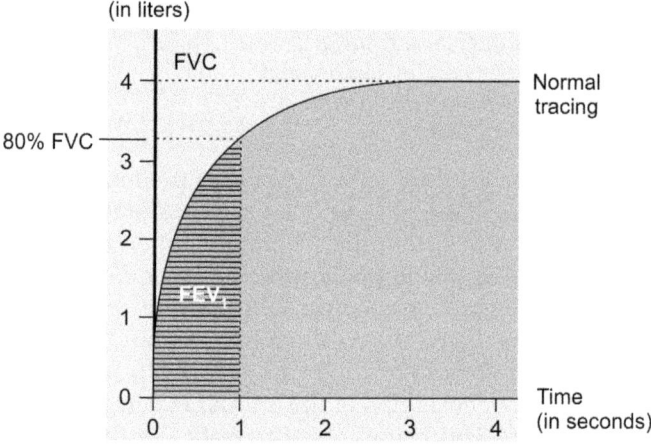

Fig. 9.2: Spirometry tracing

In restrictive lung diseases (lung fibrosis, neuromuscular problems, etc.), FVC is drastically decreased but FEV_1 is either normal or only slightly decreased. So the FEV_1/FVC ratio is more than 0.7. In obstructive lung diseases (COPD, asthma, etc.), FVC is normal or only slightly decreased but FEV_1 is drastically reduced. So, the FEV_1/FVC ratio is less than 0.7. Asthma may show the same abnormalities on spirometry as COPD. So, if there is diagnostic doubt, bronchodilator reversibility testing may be done to identify asthma.

12. What is the significance of multifocal atrial tachycardia?

Multifocal atrial tachycardia (MAT) is a cardiac arrhythmia caused by multiple sites of competing atrial activity. MAT most often is found in the elderly patient with decompensated chronic lung disease. It is thought of as a complication of underlying cardiac conduction pathology due to hypoxia. However, other underlying causes, such as heart failure, sepsis or methylxanthine toxicity may also be present (Fig. 9.3).

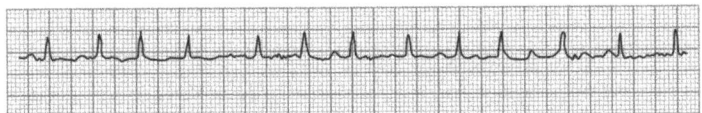

Fig. 9.3: Electrocardiography showing MAT

MAT is characterized by an irregular atrial rate greater than 100 beats per minute with atleast **3** morphologically distinct P waves, varying P-P and R-R intervals and an isoelectric baseline between the P waves. Treatment or reversal of the precipitating cause may be all that is required for patients with MAT.

13. What are the typical electrocardiographic changes observed in a patient with COPD?

The typical ECG changes seen in a patient with chronic obstructive pulmonary disease include the following (Fig. 9.4):

- Prominent tall P waves (more than 2.5 mm tall) in leads II, III and aVF, called as the P—pulmonale
- Rightward shift of the QRS axis in the frontal plane
- Poor progression of the R wave in the precordial leads
- Low voltage of the QRS complexes, especially in the left precordial leads
- The 'lead I sign'

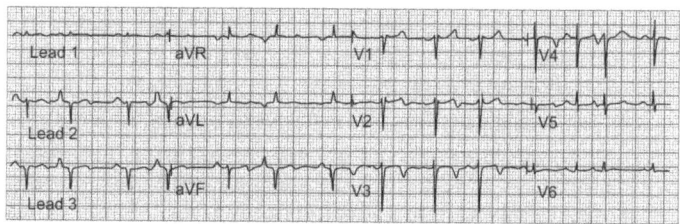

Fig. 9.4: Electrocardiographic changes in COPD

In patients with COPD and cor pulmonale, poor 'r' wave progression and the loss of R waves in right sided and mid precordial leads may sometimes mimic anterior wall myocardial infarction. Sometimes abnormal Q waves may appear in the inferior leads to suggest an inferior wall myocardial infarction. These ECG changes are usually secondary to the vertical displacement of the heart due to the low lying flattened diaphragms and the intervention of hyperinflated lungs. If the ECG recordings are taken one intercostal space lower, then the morphology of the QRS forces can be partially normalized.

14. What is the lead 1 sign?

In patients with COPD, the frontal plane P wave, QRS complex and T wave axis are all sometimes directed at around + 90 degrees. These three vectors are therefore directed either precisely or almost perpendicular to the standard lead I axis (Fig. 9.5).

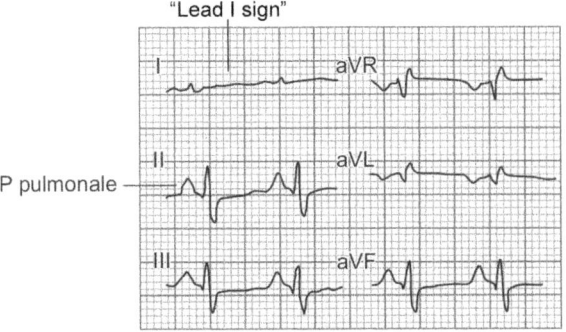

Fig. 9.5: ECG showing lead I sign

As a result of this, lead I shows either absent or very low amplitude P wave, QRS complex and T wave. This gives the appearance of a minimally disturbed baseline or an almost flat tracing in the ECG recording. This ECG phenomenon is known as the "lead I sign".

Chapter 10

Radiology

1. **What are the parameters that define a technically adequate chest chest X-ray?**

   X-rays are short wavelengths of electromagnetic radiation that penetrate matter. A radiograph is created when X-rays penetrate an object and produce an image on photographic film. The technical quality of any film must be evaluated before beginning its interpretation. Evaluation of the following five technical parameters will help to determine the technical adequacy of a chest radiograph (Table 10.1).

\<td colspan="2"\> Table 10.1: Five technically adequate parameters of chest X-ray	
Factor	**Characteristic of a technically adequate frontal chest X-ray**
1. Penetration	Thoracic spine should only be faintly seen through the heart shadow in an adequately penetrated film Too much black (i.e. overpenetrated) or too much white (i.e. underpenetrated) films may hide lesions
2. Degree of inspiration	Should see at least 5–7 anterior ribs or 8–9 posterior ribs above the midpoint of the diaphragm

   Contd...

Contd...

3. Rotation	The medial ends of the clavicles should be equidistant from the spinous process of the thoracic vertebral body in between the two clavicles
4. Projection	In a PA chest radiograph (i.e. one obtained by the posteroanterior projection), the heart being an anterior structure, is closer to the imaging surface, and thus, is truer to its actual size In an AP chest radiograph (i.e. one obtained by anteroposterior projection), the heart is farther from the imaging surface, and is therefore, slightly magnified
5. Angulation	The clavicle should have an 'S' shape and it should superimpose on the 3rd or 4th posterior ribs

2. What are the pitfalls of interpreting a technically inadequate chest X-ray?

The common pitfalls of interpreting a chest X-ray that is technically inadequate include the following (Box 10.1):

Box 10.1: Pitfalls in chest X-ray interpretation

Penetration
- The left hemidiaphragm may not be visible on an underpenetrated film because the left lung base may appear opaque
- The pulmonary markings may appear more prominent than they really are on an underpenetrated film
- The pulmonary markings may seem decreased or absent on a too dark or overpenetrated film

Inspiration
- A poor inspiratory effort will compress and crowd the lung markings, especially at the lung bases.
- A poor inspiratory effort will falsely magnify the heart

Contd...

Contd...

> **Rotation**
> - The hilum may appear large on a rotated film
> - The hemidiaphragm may appear higher on a rotated film
> - Will cause asymmetric density of lungs (i.e. one side will be darker)
>
> **Projection**
> - The heart will appear slightly larger on a film taken by anteroposterior or AP projection (portable bedside chest X-rays are always AP)
>
> **Angulation**
> - Angling the X-ray beam towards the patient's head (i.e. angulation) produces the so called apical lordotic view of the chest. This causes the clavicles to lose their normal 'S' shape and they appear straightened
> - The heart may have an abnormal shape which may some times mimic cardiomegaly

The problem of angulation occurs in hospitalized patients who may not be able to sit completely upright in bed. This causes the X-ray beam to enter the thoracic region with the patient's head and chest tilted backward. This has the effect of angling the X-ray beam towards the patient's head.

3. **How will you differentiate between anterior and posterior ribs on a frontal chest X-ray?**

   When interpreting a chest X-ray, it is important to identify the anterior and posterior ribs correctly. The following points will help in this process (Box 10.2 and Fig. 10.1).

> **Box 10.2:** Comparison between anterior and posterior ribs
>
> **Posterior ribs**
> - Are immediately more apparent to the eye
> - Are oriented more or less horizontally
> - Each pair of posterior ribs attaches to a thoracic vertebral body

Contd...

Contd...

> **Anterior ribs**
> - Are visible, but are more difficult to see
> - Are oriented downwards towards the feet
> - Attach to the sternum or to each other with cartilage that is usually not visible until later in life when the cartilage may calcify

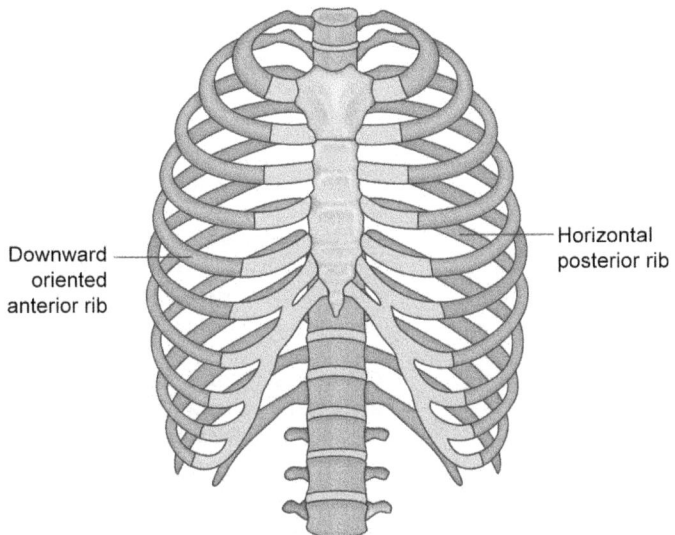

Fig. 10.1: Anterior versus posterior rib

4. **How will you systematically read a PA chest X-ray?**
   Systematic analysis of a technically adequate chest X-ray is very important to diagnose subtle anomalies. A simple method to systematically analyse a posteroanterior chest X-ray without missing any abnormality is to follow the "A,B,C,D,E,F,G,H,I" order as follows (Table 10.2):

Table 10.2: Systematic analysis of chest X-ray

Airway	• Is the airway patent and situated in the midline?
Bones	• Look for fractures, lesions, defects, osteopenia, lytic or blastic areas, erosions, lucent or sclerotic lesions
Cardiac Silhouette	• Calculate the cardiothoracic ratio (CTR) to rule out cardiomegaly • 1/3 of heart should be to the right of center • 2/3 of heart should be to the left of center
Diaphragm	• The right hemidiaphragm is normally higher than the left (the left hemidiaphragm is pushed down by the heart) • Flattened diaphragm—emphysema • Raised diaphragm—diaphragmatic paralysis, liver abscess, etc. • Gas under the diaphragm—intestinal perforation • Chilaiditi's sign—due to interposition of the large bowel between the liver and the right hemidiaphragm
Edge of the heart	• Radiopacity obscuring the heart's border—the Silhouette sign • Straightening of the left heart border—left atrial enlargement • Double density on the right heart border—left atrial enlargement
Fields of the lung	• Look for symmetry, penetration, vascularity, masses, fluid, nodules, infiltrations, bronchial cuffing, etc.
Gastric bubble	• Is the gastric air bubble obscured or absent or on the right side?

Contd...

Contd...

Hilum of the lung	• The left hilum is normally higher than the right hilum • Look for nodes or masses in the hila of both lungs
Instrumentation	• Look for any tubes, IV lines, ECG leads, surgical drains, prosthesis or other devices

5. What is the difference between PA and AP chest X-ray?

In a PA chest X-ray, the X-ray beam is fired from behind the patient and the X-ray film is placed in front of the patient. In an AP chest X-ray, the X-ray machine firing the X-ray beam is in front of the patient and the X-ray film at the back. The standard chest X-ray is PA view, but many emergency X-rays are AP. This is because AP view can be taken more easily with the patient in bed. The usual indication for an AP view film is a severely ill patient who is confined to bed (Fig. 10.2).

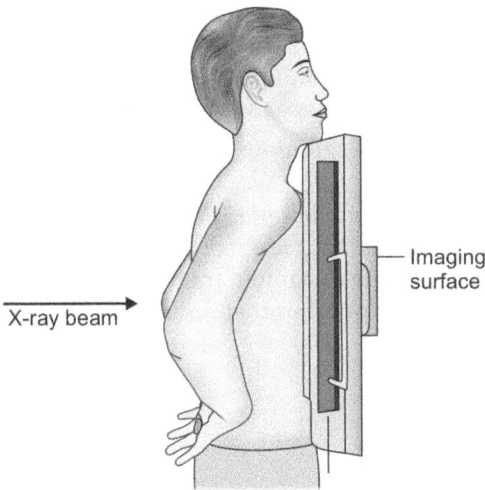

Fig. 10.2: Standard posteroanterior or PA projection

In a chest X-ray obtained by AP projection, the scapulae and the lung fields overlap. But in a PA projection (i.e. PA view) the scapulae stays clear of the lung fields (Fig. 10.3).

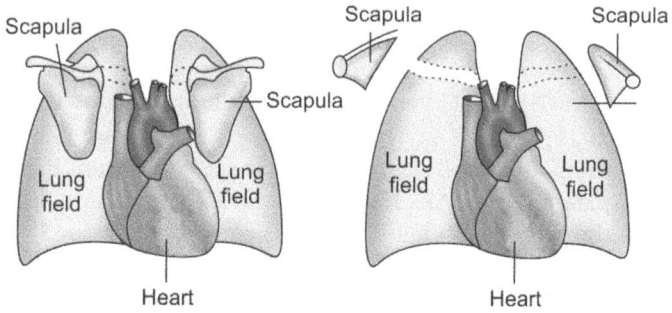

Fig. 10.3: AP versus PA view

In an AP projection, the heart is farther away from the X-ray film in the imaging cassette. Hence, there is greater magnification of the heart on the AP film. This is called as pseudocardiomegaly. Another common cause for pseudocardiomegaly is an expiratory chest X-ray.

6. **How will you calculate cardiothoracic ratio on the chest X-ray?**
   The cardiothoracic ratio (CTR) on the PA chest X-ray gives an idea about the size of the heart. It is obtained by dividing the maximum transverse cardiac silhouette by the maximum internal thoracic diameter as shown in Figure 10.4.

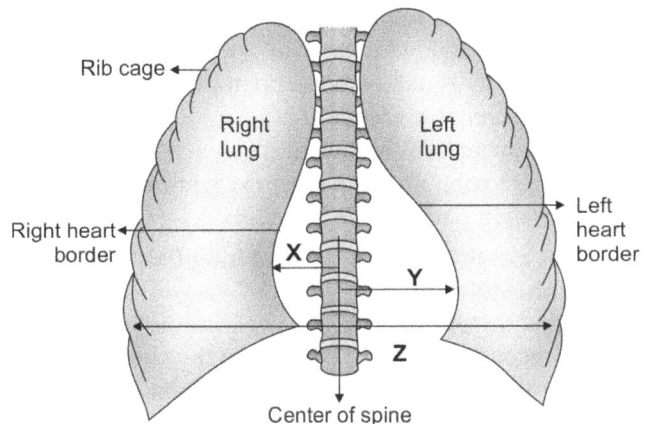

Fig. 10.4: Calculation of cardiothoracic ratio

$$\text{Cardiothoracic ratio} = \frac{X + Y}{Z}$$

X = Maximum distance from the center of spine to the right border of heart

Y = Maximum distance from the center of spine to the left border of heart

Z = Maximum internal thoracic diameter

In people with normal sized heart, the cardiothoracic ratio is usually less than 50%. In those with cardiomegaly, the cardiothoracic ratio is more than 50%. A heart may have higher (i.e. more than 50%) cardiothoracic ratio and still be a normal heart. This can occur if there is an extracardiac cause of cardiac enlargement. Extracardiac

causes producing cardiomegaly on the chest X-ray include the following:
- Inability to take a deep breath because of obesity, pregnancy or ascites
- Abnormalities of the chestwall that compresses the heart such as the pectus excavatum deformity or straight back syndrome.

7. What are the various types of lung field shadows on the chest X-ray?

Most of the diseases have a specific radiological pattern and recognition of this pattern on the chest X-ray is an important diagnostic clue. Lung field shadows are of the following important types.
- Nodular shadows—in military tuberculosis, metastasis, adenoma etc.
- Reticular shadows (network of fine lines)—in fibrosis
- Reticulonodular shadows—in interstitial lung disease
- Alveolar shadows—in pneumonia, left ventricular failure, ARDS, etc.
- Ring shadows—in cavitating lesions, bronchiectasis, etc.
- Linear shadows—Kerley's B lines in early pulmonary edema (due to prominent interlobular lymphatics).

8. What are the things that should be carefully looked for in an apparently normal chest X-ray?

In an apparently normal looking chest x-ray, one should carefully look for the following findings which are otherwise usually overlooked (Fig. 10.5):
- Small apical pneumothorax
- Cervical rib
- Rib pathology like fracture, notching or metastatic infiltration
- Air under the diaphragm (in perforated viscus)
- Double left heart border (in left lower lobe collapse)

- Paravertebral abscess (in tuberculosis of the spine)
- Foreign body in the trachea
- Double density on right heart border (in left atrial dilatation)

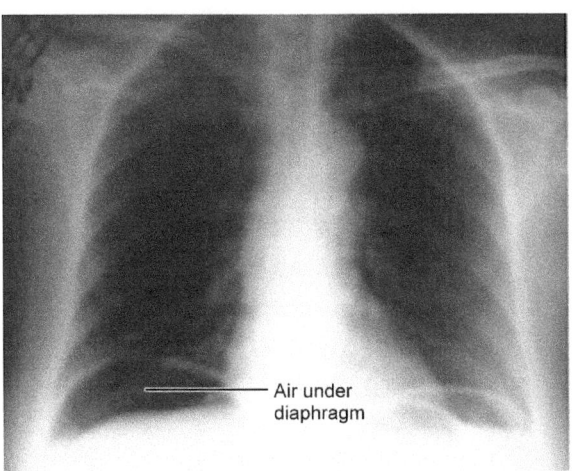

Fig. 10.5: X-ray in intestinal perforation

9. **What are the features of hyperinflation on the chest x-ray?**

   Hyperinflation is a feature seen in obstructive airway diseases like COPD, and it has the following features (Fig. 10.6):
   - Only up to the anterior end of the 6th rib or upto the posterior 10th rib should be visible above the diaphragm. If more ribs are visible, then there is hyperinflation
   - Tubular heart (due to the overexpansion of the rib cage)
   - Flat hemidiaphragms
   - Large central pulmonary arteries
   - Decreased peripheral vascular markings
   - Bullae may be present (may mimic pneumothorax)

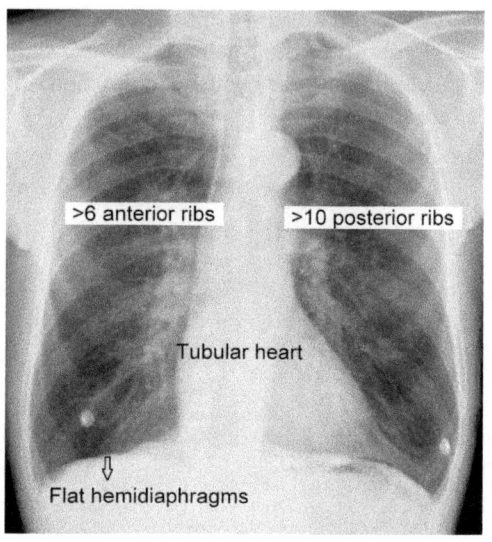

Fig. 10.6: X-ray showing hyperinflation

10. What is the role of chest X-ray in pleural effusion?

The pleural fluid first accumulates in the most dependent portion of the thoracic cavity which is the posterior costophrenic sulcus or angle. Therefore, the earliest radiological sign of a pleural effusion is the blunting of the posterior costophrenic angle on the lateral chest radiograph (Fig. 10.7). In a standard upright chest X-ray, it takes only about 75 mL of fluid to blunt the posterior costophrenic angle on the lateral view film. However, 250–300 mL of fluid is required to blunt the lateral costophrenic angles on a frontal (PA or AP) film (*Ref: The Washington Manual of Medical Therapeutics, 33rd edition*).

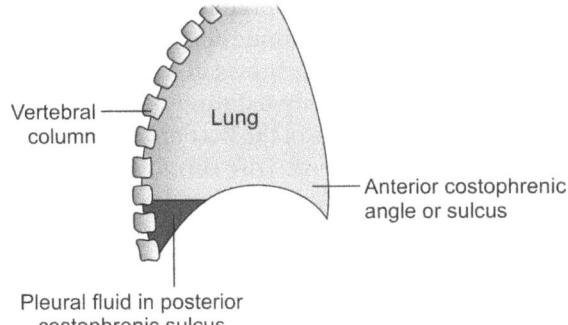

Fig. 10.7: Lateral view chest X-ray in pleural effusion

Chest X-ray lateral decubitus view demonstrates fluidity and can demonstrate as little as 25–50 mL of pleural fluid (*Ref: Fishman's Pulmonary Diseases* 4th *edition,* Pg 457*)*. USG is more sensitive in diagnosing minimal effusion and subpulmonic effusion.

11. What is the most important sign of consolidation on the chest X-ray?

The air bronchogram sign is the most definite sign of consolidation of lung tissue. This sign may be seen in atelectasis also. Air bronchogram sign is the radiographic shadow of an air-filled bronchus (i.e. a radiolucent area) running through an airless area of lung (i.e. an opacified area).

On a normal radiograph, the bronchi are not normally visible unless seen end on. In consolidation, the air in the alveoli is replaced with inflammatory exudates which later on solidify. So, these alveolar areas may be seen as an opacified area. The air-filled bronchi passing through the same opacified area may be visible as branching linear lucencies, or air bronchograms.

12. What is "silhouette" sign?

"Silhouette" sign is an important radiological sign. There are actually four radiographic densities. They are (1) air, (2) fat, (3) bone and (4) water/soft tissue. A clear border is seen radiologically only at the interface of two different densities as in the case of the border between heart (i.e. water) and lung (i.e. air). This 'silhouette' is lost if air in the lung is replaced by consolidated or collapsed airless solidified lung tissue. This is the "silhouette" sign and it helps in localizing middle lobe pathologies like middle lobe consolidation or collapse (Fig. 10.8).

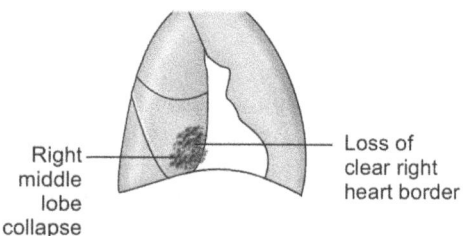

Fig. 10.8: Positive silhouette sign

13. What is hilum overlay sign?

Hilum overlay sign helps to differentiate an enlarged pulmonary artery from a mediastinal mass in the hilar region overlying the large central pulmonary vessels. The demonstration of pulmonary vessels converging medial to the apparent lateral margin of the "mass" indicates that it is not the artery that is enlarged. The converse (i.e. the hilum convergence sign), suggest that, when pulmonary vessels converge to the lateral margin of an apparent hilar "mass" like shadow, then the "mass" that is enlarged is the pulmonary artery itself.

14. What is the importance of measuring the right descending pulmonary artery on a chest X-ray?

The right descending pulmonary artery or RDPA is visible on all chest X-rays as a large descending vessel just to the right of the right heart border. Its diameter can be measured at about the level of the indentation between the ascending aorta and the right atrium. In normal people, the RDPA is less than 17 mm in diameter. In pulmonary venous or arterial hypertension, the RDPA is usually greater than 17 mm in diameter.

15. What do the terms "cephalization" and "pruning" mean with respect to pulmonary hypertension?

Cephalization is the term used to denote that the upper lobe blood vessels are equal to or greater than the size of the lower lobe blood vessels. Cephalization is a feature of pulmonary venous hypertension.

Pruning means that there is a rapid decrease in the size of the peripheral blood vessels relative to the central vessels from which they come. Pruning is a feature of pulmonary arterial hypertension.

16. What are the characteristics of a benign solitary pulmonary nodule?

A solitary pulmonary nodule (SPN/coin lesion) is a less than 3 cm size rounded opacity on the chest radiograph. It is outlined by normal lung parenchyma and is not associated with other infiltrates, atelectasis or adenopathy. Most are asymptomatic but the finding is important because it carries a significant risk of malignancy.

Common causes for SPN include carcinoma of the lung (15–50%), fungal infections, tuberculosis, uncalcified granulomas, resolving pneumonia, hamartoma and metastatic lesions. The following are the important features that help to differentiate a benign SPN from a malignant SPN (Table 10.3).

Table 10.3: Differentiation between benign SPN and malignant SPN

Clinical parameter	Benign SPN	Malignant SPN
Age	Less than 30 years	More than 30 years
Smoking	No	Yes
Nodule size	Less than 2 cms	More than 2 cms
Nodule age or duration	More than 2 years	Less than 2 years
Nodule doubling time	Less than 30 days in infective benign lesions More than 365 days in other benign lesions	Usually 30 to 365 days
Nodule margins	Smooth	Irregular
Presence of calcification	Yes (central or laminated)	Rare

17. What are the features that help to differentiate pulmonary edema due to ARDS from hydrostatic pulmonary edema on a chest X-ray?

Hydrostatic pulmonary edema is usually caused by cardiac failure or fluid overload states. ALI (acute lung injury) and ARDS (acute respiratory distress syndrome) usually produces non-hydrostatic permeability edema. The American European Consensus Conference (AECC) has defined both ALI and ARDS. ALI requires all four of the following features in patients who have a risk factor for ARDS (like septicemia) and no history of chronic lung disease.

- Acute onset
- Bilateral lung infiltrates
- No evidence of elevated left atrial pressure (the pulmonary capillary wedge pressure is ≤18 mm Hg)

- A ratio of arterial oxygen tension to fraction of inspired oxygen (i.e. PaO_2/FiO_2) of 201 to 300 mm Hg.

Definition of ARDS is the same, except that the PaO_2/FiO_2 ratio is ≤ 200 mm Hg. The radiological features that help to differentiate between the two types of pulmonary edema are the following (Table 10.4):

Table 10.4: Differences between hydrostatic and permeability edema

Hydrostatic edema (cardiac failure)	Permeability edema (ALI, ARDS)
Symmetric and diffuse opacity	Asymmetric and patchy opacity
Perihilar distribution	Peripheral distribution
Kerley B lines present	Usually absent
Vascular redistribution present	Usually absent
Cardiomegaly present	Usually absent
Pleural effusion may be present	Usually absent

18. How will you distinguish between a giant bullae and pneumothorax on a plain radiograph of the chest?

Giant bullae may simulate the radiographic appearance of pneumothorax. On plain chest radiographs, the characteristics of the visceral pleural line help to differentiate a giant, thin-walled bulla from a pneumothorax.

The presence of a pneumothorax is established by demonstrating a white visceral pleural line on the chest radiograph. The visceral pleural line defines the interface of the lung and pleural air. In general, the pleural line associated with a large bulla is usually concave (i.e. open angle) relative to the lateral chest wall, whereas the pleural line associated with a pneumothorax is either convex (i.e. narrow angle) or straight relative to the lateral chest wall. However, the two conditions are more easily differentiated by computed tomography of the chest (Fig. 10.9).

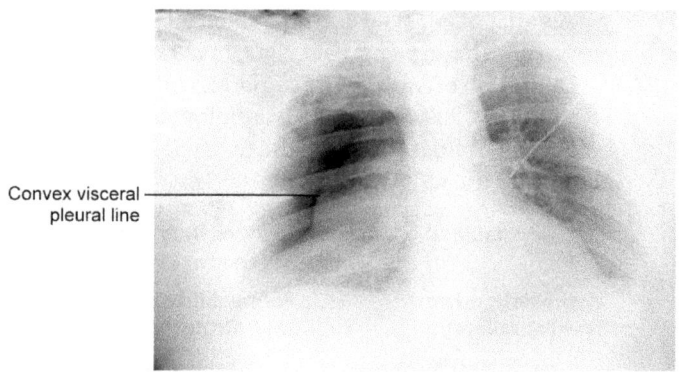

Fig. 10.9: Visceral pleural line in pneumothorax

19. What is vanishing lung syndrome?

Vanishing lung syndrome is a radiological syndrome in which the lungs appear to be disappearing on the chest X-ray. The syndrome is characterized by a progressive decrease in the radiographic opacity of the lung. Causes of vanishing lung syndrome include the accelerated progression of emphysema destroying the lung or the rapid cystic destruction of the lung by infection.

Index

Page numbers followed by *f* refer to figure and *t* refer to table.

A

Abscess
   metastatic 121
   paravertebral 155
   subdiaphragmatic 67
Acid-fast bacilli 115
Adenomas 7
Adson's test 62
Adventitious sounds 84*t*
Airflow limitation, severe 15
Airway 150
   obstruction, acute 3
Allergic bronchopulmonary
   aspergillosis 121-123
   mycoses 102
Alveolar exudate, eosinophilic 130
Amebiasis, pulmonary 9
American College of Chest
   Physicians 84
American European Consensus
   Conference 160
American Thoracic Society
   Committee 85
Amphoric bronchial breath
   sound 83
Amyloidosis, secondary 121
Anemia, hemolytic 131
Anorexia 130
Antibiotics 130
Antituberculosis treatment 109
Arteries, bronchial 8
Arteriovenous shunting,
   intrapulmonary 141
Arthritis 37
Asbestosis 98, 100
Ascites 80
Aspergilloma 6, 7
Aspergillus 133
   clavatus 103
   fumigatus 123
Aspiration 117
   recurrent 130
   role of 131
Asterixis 30
   causes of 30
Asthma 10, 60, 86, 123, 137, 138*t*
   bronchial 4, 15, 16, 16*t*
   cardiac 15, 16
   cough variant 14
   intrinsic 137
   occupational 15
   refractory 137
Atelectasis 50, 116
   recurrent 121
Atenolol 35
Atrial tachycardia, multifocal 143
Axillary lymph nodes 33
Azoospermia, obstructive 121

B

Barrel-shaped chest 44*f*, 45
  peculiarity of 44
Berylliosis 100, 118
Biot's respiration 39
Blood
  flow, pulmonary 141
  gas analysis, arterial 25
  pressure 31
  vessels 8
    walls of 8
  viscosity 141
Body cavity 74
Bones 150
Bornholm disease 1
Breast cancer 56
Breath sound 54*f*, 79, 79*f*, 92
  bronchial 55*f*, 81, 81*f*, 81*t*
Breathing
  peculiarities of 99
  types of 46
Brock's syndrome 117, 121
Bronchial
  asthma, severe 32
  breath sounds, types of 82
Bronchiectasis 5, 7, 117, 119-121, 124, 124*f*
  complications of 121
  cystic 95
  infective exacerbations of 123
Bronchitis, chronic 3, 4, 9, 122
Bronchodilators 16
Broncholithiasis 117
Bronchopneumonia 125
Bronchorrhea 54
Bronchoscopy 133
Bruton agammaglobulinemia 121
Bucket handle movement 45

C

Calcareous masses,
    dislodgement of 8
Campbell's sign 47
Cancer, colon 56
Cannon-ball lesions 56
Capillary permeability 68
Caplan's syndrome 101
Captopril 35
Carbamazepine 35
Carbon dioxide narcosis 30
Carcinomas 7
Cardiopulmonary disease,
    primary 141
Cardiothoracic ratio,
    calculation of 153*f*
Carpopedal spasm 41
Catamenial pneumothorax 75
Cavernous bronchial breath
    sound 83
Cavitary lung disease 7
Cavitation, pulmonary 116
Cellophane crackles 89
Centriacinar emphysema 14
Cephalosporins 35
Cerebrospinal fluid 113
Chest
  auscultation of 79
  drain 73
  pain 54, 80
    pleuritic 1
  percussion 59, 60*f*
  tube insertion 73
  wall 54*f*
    pain 1
    palpation of 43
    tumor infiltration of 18
  X-ray 130, 146*t*, 155
    interpretation 147
    systematic analysis of 150*t*

Cheyne-Stokes respiration 39
Chlamydia pneumoniae 130
Choriocarcinoma 56
Churg-Strauss syndrome 101, 102, 118
Chvostek's sign 41
Ciliary dyskinesia, primary 120
Circulatory collapse syndrome 11
Cirrhosis 68
    biliary 25
Clubbing 20, 89
    causes of 24, 25
    mechanism of 20
Coal worker's pneumoconiosis 98, 100
Cobb's angle 45, 46f
Collagen vascular disease 98
Collar stud abscesses 32
Community-acquired pneumonia 126, 127
Compression collapse 51, 52f
Conjunctivitis, phlyctenular 36
Cor pulmonale 29, 30, 30t, 121, 123, 140, 141
Corticosteroid 109
Costochondritis 18, 19, 19t
    syndrome 19
Cough 16, 90
    chronic 4, 37
    nonproductive 130
    postural 4
    syncope 5
Coxiella burnetti 130
Coxsackie B virus infection 1
Cracked-pot resonance 66
C-reactive protein 114
Crohn's disease 25
Curb score calculation 127f
Cyanosis 14, 25, 28, 29f
    central 26, 26t, 89
    peripheral 26, 26t, 27f
Cystic fibrosis, complications of 123
Cysts
    congenital 95
    traumatic 95
Cytomegalovirus 133

D

D'Espine's sign 82
Dialysis dementia 30
Diaphragm 150
Diaphragmatic tumors, neurogenic 25
Directly observed treatment, short-course 112
Distal phalangeal depth 22
Drug reactions, adverse 116
Dry bronchiectasis 120
Dyspnea 9, 12, 16
    acute onset of 10
    onset of 10
    syndrome 11

E

Ectopic abscess formation 131
Edema 99
    hydrostatic 161
        pulmonary 160
    pulmonary 160
    re-expansion pulmonary 70
Egophony 96
Electrocardiography 11, 143
Embolism, pulmonary 3, 10
Emphysema 3, 60, 141
    types of 14t

Empyema 72, 73, 116, 121, 131
- formation 130
- necessitans 19

Encephalopathy, hepatic 30
Endocarditis, infective 25
Eosinophilia 102
Eosinophilic pneumonia
- acute 102
- chronic 102

Epstein-Barr virus 34
Erythema nodosum 36
Erythrocyte sedimentation rate 34, 114
Esophagus, rupture of 67
Ewart's sign 66, 66*f*
Exudative, types of 69

F

Facial plethora 28
Farmer's lung disease 103
Fever 110
- moderate grade 130

Fibrosis 93*f*, 99, 116
- cystic 12, 25, 122, 123
- interstitial 99
- pulmonary 92

Fibrothorax 49
Filariasis 102
Fistula, bronchopleural 84
Flexible bronchoscopy 133
Floating nail sign 21
Fungal infections 95, 118, 120
Fungi 6, 133

G

Ganglioneuroma 83
Garland's triangle 66
Gastric bubble 150
Gastroesophageal reflux 4
- disease 137

Ghon's complex 105
Ghon's focus 106
Giant bullae 161
Goodpasture's syndrome 101
Granuloma formation 118
Granulomatous pulmonary diseases 118
Grave's disease 25
Grocco's and Garland's triangle 65, 65*f*

H

Haemophilus influenzae 121
Heart
- diseases, cyanotic congenital 25
- edge of 150
- failure 68
- rate 31

Hematemesis 5, 5*t*
Hemoptysis 5, 5*t*, 6, 7, 110, 121, 123
- recurrent 7
- syndrome 11

Hepatojugular reflex 30
Hepatopulmonary syndrome 141
Hernias, inguinal 37
Hilum overlay sign 158
HIV infection 109
Hoover's sign 48
Horner's syndrome 53
Hospital-acquired pneumonia 127
Hydatid cyst 95
Hydropneumothorax 95
Hydrothorax, hepatic 67
Hypercalcemia 55
Hypercapnia 3
- mixed 4
- severe 139
- signs of 4

Hyperemia, conjunctival 4
Hypereosinophilic syndrome 102
Hyperinflation 155, 156*f*
Hyperpnea 38
Hypertension 4
    pulmonary 159
Hypertrophy 29
Hyperventilation syndrome 12, 40, 41
Hypokalemia 30
Hypomagnesemia 30
Hypoproteinemia 121
Hypothalamic-pituitary-adrenal axis 136
Hypoventilation
    severe 4
    syndrome, congenital central 40
Hypoxemia 3, 4, 25
    arterial 141
Hypoxia, alveolar 141

I

Idiopathic pulmonary fibrosis 98
Infarction 7
    pulmonary 95
Infection 133
    chronic 139
    pulmonary 9
Inflammation 117
Injury, causes of 18
Intercostal muscles, severe myalgia of 1
Internal ring 36*f*
Interphalangeal depth 22
Interstitial lung disease, causes of 98
Interstitium 130
Intestinal perforation 155*f*
Intracardiac shunt 3
Intradermal tuberculin protein 108*f*

K

Kaposi's sarcoma 6
Kartagener's syndrome 120
Kerley's B lines 154, 161
Kikuchi's disease 34
    signs 34
    symptoms 34
Kikuchi's histiocytic necrotizing lymphadenitis 34
Kikuchi-Fujimoto disease 34
Klebsiella pneumoniae 9
Kronig's isthmus 61, 61*f*
Kyphosis 45, 46*f*
    severity of 45

L

Lactate dehydrogenase 68
Lambert-Eaton syndrome 55
Laryngeal nerve recurrent 17, 17*f*, 18
Laryngitis 16
Latent tuberculosis infection 105
Legionella pneumophila 130
Leukemia 109
Light's criteria 68
Litten's sign 53
Liver disease 111, 141
Lobar collapse 50, 123
Loffler's syndrome 102
Lovibond's angle 21, 21*f*
Lumen obstruction, bronchial 119
Lung
    abscess 25, 95, 121, 131
    cancer 25
    cavity 95

collapse of 54f
disease 5, 37
    interstitial 3, 12, 25, 89, 98, 99, 101, 120
    restrictive 143
fibrosis 143
fields of 150
hilum of 151
lobes 50, 56
    collapse of 54
    types of 57t
malignancy 55
Lymph node
    excision 32
    mediastinal 106
Lymphadenopathy 32, 35
    intrathoracic 116
Lymphedema 121
Lymphocyte predominant pleural effusion 121
Lymphoma 50, 109

M

Macrophages 118
Malaise 130
Malignancy, bronchogenic 50
Mantoux method 107
Marfan syndrome 43
Mass, abdominal 80
Mediastinal lymphadenopathy, causes of 50
Meigs' syndrome 67
Melanoma 56
Melanoptysis 6
Mendelson's syndrome 132
Metastases, pulmonary 56
Miliary disease 116
Mucus 8
Multiple drug resistant tuberculosis 111

Myalgia
    epidemic 1
    syndrome 102
Mycobacterial infections 118
Mycobacterium tuberculosis 105, 107
Mycoplasma 137
    pneumoniae 130, 131
Myoclonus 4

N

Nails, yellow-green discoloration of 121
Nasal polyps 123
Necrobiotic nodule 101
Nephrotic syndrome 68
Neurofibroma 83
Neurogenic thoracic outlet syndrome 62
Neuromuscular disorders 3
Noninvasive positive pressure ventilation 139

O

Obesity hypoventilation syndrome 85
Obstruction, bronchial 130
Obstructive
    collapse 51
    lung disease, chronic 139
    pulmonary disease, chronic 134
Oliver's sign 48
Ondine's curse 40
Open-negative syndrome 115
Orthopnea 12

P

Pain
    pleuritic 1, 11
    sensation, pathways of 2

Panacinar emphysema 14
Pancoast syndrome 62
Pancoast tumor 61
Pancreatitis, acute onset of 67
Papilledema 4
Paraneoplastic syndromes 53, 55
Parapneumonic effusion 131
Parasitic infestations 102
Parenchymal lesion, primary 106
Paroxysmal nocturnal dyspnea 9
Patent ductus arteriosus 28
Patent tuberculosis 104
Pectus deformities 43
Pectus excavatum 43
Penicillin 35
Peribronchial nodes 120
Pericarditis, purulent 121
Phantom tumor 69
Phenytoin 35
Phlegm 8
Phrenic nerve infiltration 53
Pickwickian syndrome 85
PIE syndrome 102
Pigeon chest 43
Platelet-derived growth factor 21
Platypnea 12
Pleurodynia 1
Pneumoconiosis 98, 99, 100*t*
Pneumocystis aureus 131
Pneumocystis jirovecii 130, 131, 133
   pneumonia 130
Pneumonia 3, 11, 125, 129, 131, 132
   acute onset of 122
   atypical 130
   interstitial 125, 130
   lipoid 132
   lobar 9, 125, 128
   nonresolving 54, 129, 130
   recurrent 121
   types of 126*f*
Pneumonitis, hypersensitivity 102, 118
Pneumothorax 5, 10, 58, 60*f*, 75, 80, 131, 161, 162*f*
Poisons 10
Polycythemia 141
   vera 28
Polymyositis 101
Poncet's disease 36
Postnasal drip syndrome 4
Post-tussive suction 93
   sound 83, 94*f*
Precordial catch syndrome 2
Progressive massive fibrosis 6
Pseudobronchiectasis 122
Pseudoclubbing 24
Pseudomonas aeruginosa 6
Pulsus paradoxus 32
Pump
   failure 10
   handle movement 38*f*, 45
Pyrazinamide 111

Q

Quinidine 35

R

Rasmussen aneurysm 116
   rupture of 8
Raynaud's phenomenon 62
Recurrent small pulmonary emboli 7
Renal cell carcinoma 56
Resistant organisms 130
Respiration 39*f*
Respiratory
   acidosis, severe 139

diseases 32
failure 2, 123
    types of 3t
muscle weakness 80
pump 4
system 12, 84, 97
Reticulonodular shadows 154
Rheumatic disorders 101, 101t
Rheumatoid
    arthritis 98, 101
    nodule 101
Rhinosinusitis 137
Ribs
    anterior 148, 149, 149f
    cervical 62, 154
    fracture 5, 18
    pathology 154
    posterior 148, 149f
Rifampin 111
Right middle lobe syndrome 121
Ring shadows 154

S

Sarcoidosis 33, 50, 98, 118
Scalene lymph node, palpation of 33f
Schamroth's sign 22, 22f
Scleroderma 101
Scoliosis 46
Shrinking lungs 98
    syndrome 100
Sickle-cell disease 141
Silhouette sign 158, 158f
Silicosis 98, 100, 118
Simple pulmonary eosinophilia 102
Sinopulmonary infections, chronic 121
Sinus arrhythmia 31f, 32
Sinusitis 120
Situs inversus 120
Sjögren's syndrome 101
Small apical pneumothorax 154
Small cell lung cancer 53, 55
Solitary pulmonary nodule, benign 159
Spermatogenesis, normal 121
Spirometry tracing 142f
Spontaneous pneumothorax 123
    types of 74
Sputum, color of 9, 9t
Squamous cell
    carcinoma 95
    lung cancer 55
    tumor 62
Staphylococcus aureus 122, 127, 131
Staphylococcus pneumoniae 127
Stomach, herniation of 95
Stridor 84
Strongyloides 102
Sulfonamides 35, 102
Superior vena cava
    obstruction 30, 30t, 53
    syndrome 29, 53
Sweating 110
Sympathetic chain infiltration 53
Systemic lupus erythematosus 98

T

T lymphocytes 118
Tachycardia 4
Tachypnea 4
Tactile fremitus 58
Tension pneumothorax 75
Testicular teratomas 56
Thermophilic actinomycetes 103

Thiazides 102
Thoracic
  cavity 95
  endometriosis syndrome 75
  outlet syndrome 62
Thyroid
  acropachy 25
  cancer 56
Tietze's syndrome 18, 19, 19*t*
Tracheal tug 48
Transudative pleural effusions 69
Traube's area 63, 64*f*
Trepopnea 12
Troisier's sign 33
Trousseau's sign 41
  elicitation of 41*f*
Tuberculin test 116
Tuberculosis 5, 50, 61, 95, 100, 104, 110, 112, 117, 120, 121
  extrapulmonary 113
  post-primary 106, 116, 116*t*
  primary 36, 106*f*
  pulmonary 4, 7, 8, 107, 115
  treatment of 112
Tuberculous
  cavity 96
  infection, primary 104*f*
  pleural effusion 70-72
  rheumatism 36
Tubular bronchial breath sound 82, 93*f*, 128*f*
Tumors
  benign 117
  bronchial 7, 86
  lymphatic 83
  malignant 117

U

Ulcerative colitis 25

Unilateral pleural effusion, non-respiratory causes of 67
Uremia 30

V

Vanishing lung syndrome 162
Vascular thoracic outlet syndrome 62
Vasculitic disorders 102
Vasoconstriction, pulmonary 141
Veins, pulmonary 8
Velcro crackles 89
Venous pressure 68
Vesicular breath sound 80, 80*f*, 81
Viral infections 109
Virchow's node 33
Viruses 130
Vocal fremitus 58

W

Waldeyer's ring 35
  adenopathy 35
Wegener's granulomatosis 95, 101, 118
Wheeze 85
  classification of 86*t*
  polyphonic 86
  production of 86*f*
  types of 86
Whispering pectoriloquy 83
Wrist joint 60*f*

Y

Yellow nail syndrome 121
Young's syndrome 121

Z

Ziehl-Neelsen staining 107

EU GSPR Authorised Reprsentative
Logos Europe, 9 rue Nicolas Poussin
1700, La Rochelle, France
Phone: +33 (0) 6 67 93 73 78
E-mail: contact@logoseurope.eu

www.ingramcontent.com/pod-product-compliance
Ingram Content Group UK Ltd.
Pitfield, Milton Keynes, MK11 3LW, UK
UKHW021829140426
5217IPUK00021B/1345